High-Fidelity
Medical Imaging
Displays

Tutorial Texts Series

High-Fidelity Medical Imaging Displays

Aldo Badano

Michael J. Flynn

Jerzy Kanicki

Tutorial Texts in Optical Engineering
Volume TT63

SPIE
PRESS

Bellingham, Washington USA

Library of Congress Cataloging-in-Publication Data

Badano, Aldo.
   High-fidelity medical imaging displays / Aldo Badano, Michael J. Flynn, Jerzy Kanicki.
      p. cm. – (Tutorial texts in optical engineering ; TT63)
   ISBN 0-8194-5191-6 (softcover)
   1. Imaging systems in medicine. 2. Liquid crystal displays. 3. Cathode ray tubes. I.
Flynn, Michael J. II. Kanicki, Jerzy. III. Title. IV. Series.

R857.O6B33 2003
616.07'54—dc22   2003056856

Published by

SPIE—The International Society for Optical Engineering
P.O. Box 10
Bellingham, Washington 98227-0010 USA
Phone: +1 360 676 3290
Fax: +1 360 647 1445
Email: spie@spie.org
Web: http://spie.org

The content of this book reflects the work and thought of the author(s).
Every effort has been made to publish reliable and accurate information herein,
but the publisher is not responsible for the validity of the information or for any
outcomes resulting from reliance thereon.

Printed in the United States of America.

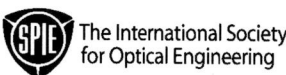
The International Society
for Optical Engineering

Introduction to the Series

Since its conception in 1989, the Tutorial Texts series has grown to more than 60 titles covering many diverse fields of science and engineering. When the series was started, the goal of the series was to provide a way to make the material presented in SPIE short courses available to those who could not attend, and to provide a reference text for those who could. Many of the texts in this series are generated from notes that were presented during these short courses. But as stand-alone documents, short course notes do not generally serve the student or reader well. Short course notes typically are developed on the assumption that supporting material will be presented verbally to complement the notes, which are generally written in summary form to highlight key technical topics and therefore are not intended as stand-alone documents. Additionally, the figures, tables, and other graphically formatted information accompanying the notes require the further explanation given during the instructor's lecture. Thus, by adding the appropriate detail presented during the lecture, the course material can be read and used independently in a tutorial fashion.

What separates the books in this series from other technical monographs and textbooks is the way in which the material is presented. To keep in line with the tutorial nature of the series, many of the topics presented in these texts are followed by detailed examples that further explain the concepts presented. Many pictures and illustrations are included with each text and, where appropriate, tabular reference data are also included.

The topics within the series have grown from the initial areas of geometrical optics, optical detectors, and image processing to include the emerging fields of nanotechnology, biomedical optics, and micromachining. When a proposal for a text is received, each proposal is evaluated to determine the relevance of the proposed topic. This initial reviewing process has been very helpful to authors in identifying, early in the writing process, the need for additional material or other changes in approach that would serve to strengthen the text. Once a manuscript is completed, it is peer reviewed to ensure that chapters communicate accurately the essential ingredients of the processes and technologies under discussion.

It is my goal to maintain the style and quality of books in the series, and to further expand the topic areas to include new emerging fields as they become of interest to our reading audience.

Arthur R. Weeks, Jr.
University of Central Florida

Contents

List of Figures

List of Tables

Preface

This book is based on a short course given by the authors at SPIE's Medical Imaging International Symposium from 1999 to 2002. During those years, the number of commercially available medical display systems increased considerably. For instance, during the 84th annual meeting of the Radiological Society of North America (RSNA) held in Chicago in 1998, three different liquid crystal prototypes were showcased on the commercial exhibit floor by just a few vendors. In the 88th RSNA meeting held in the same city in 2002, more than 20 different liquid crystal technologies in more than 100 models were present on the exhibit floor.

At the same time, we have witnessed a significant increase in the interest level of the community about display system performance and application requirements. We have also experienced an exciting feeling that this is just the beginning of a rapidly evolving story that will be nurtured by new technologies and new applications. The number of modalities that rely on the electronic presentation of image data is growing rapidly, including computed tomography, mammography, chest and bone radiography, ultrasound, and image-guided interventional procedures. Moreover, this growth has been emphasized by the availability of powerful computer networks that allow remote users to receive large image datasets and display them in their portable computers or personal digital appliances. This changing scenario also brings challenges regarding how these devices and systems are used, and about how physical measurements can be used to assess image quality. It is in this spirit that we present in this book the expanded content of the short course.

This book is organized into six chapters. Chapters 1 and 2 introduce medical imaging displays by defining the requirements for a high-fidelity display performance, and by summarizing human visual system characteristics with respect to luminance, contrast, resolution, glare, and reflection. Chapters 3 and 4 introduce the different display technologies that have, or are likely to have, an impact on medical imaging workstations today or in the future. Chapter 3 presents a review of the ubiquitous cathode-ray tube (CRT), and Chapter 4 describes the active-matrix liquid crystal display (AMLCD). Chapter 5 presents the current challenges in the development of an emerging display technology based on light-emitting organic molecules and polymer devices that will likely be present in many portable display solutions in the coming few years. Having described the requirements for a high-fidelity display and its intrinsic device properties, we develop, in Chapter 6, methods for the assessment of display image quality. In this chapter, we focus on methods that are useful to characterize display performance while allowing the measurement of image quality up to, and even beyond, the limits of the human visual system.

Most of the methods presented in this book are described in a way that clinical engineers and medical physicists can utilize them in a clinical environment as long as they have access to the appropriate instrumentation. This tutorial is not, however, a collection of ready-to-use procedures or techniques. Readers interested in more practical aspects of display quality assessment should consider the recommendations of the American Association of Physicists in Medicine (AAPM),[143] or the collection of measurement methods assembled in the Flat Panel Display Measurement Standard.[58] Our perspective in this book is to offer a more general tutorial on display image quality, its relationship to device technology, and the methodologies for its assessment. At the same time, the methods and techniques described will allow other readers who are involved in the design, manufacture, marketing, purchase, and management of displays for digital radiology systems to make informed decisions about display devices and display image quality by better understanding the device requirements and specifications.

Much of the effort in this book was supported by the Center for Devices and Radiological Health (CDRH) from the Food and Drug Administration (FDA), the National Institutes of Health (NIH), and the Defense Advanced Research Projects Agency (DARPA). I would like to express our thanks to the many reviewers of the manuscript in its various forms including Rachel Leimbach, Susan Hipper, Ben Imhoff, and Sarah Drilling—all student interns from the Department of Biomedical Engineering at Marquette University. We are also thankful for the useful discussions with Ehsan Samei (Duke University), Sandrine Martin (University of Michigan), Ken Compton (National Display Systems), Robert J. Jennings (CDRH, FDA), Robert M. Gagne (CDRH, FDA), Kyle J. Myers (CDRH, FDA), and Robert F. Wagner (CDRH, FDA) that have made this book better.

Aldo Badano
July 2004

Chapter 1
Introduction

*Display: dis·play. Pronunciation: di-'splA. Etymology:
Middle English, from Anglo-French despleer, desploier,
literally, to unfold. Date: 14th century. a: to put or spread
before the view* <display the flag>, *b: to make evident*
<displayed great skill>, *c: to exhibit ostentatiously*
<liked to display his erudition>.

— Merriam-Webster Online Dictionary

Displays are devices used for delivery of information, and as such have been used since ancient ages. Over time, display devices have been used more and more in human communication activities. However, it was not until the twentieth century that display devices capable of delivering high-information content became a necessity as well as a reality for many applications. In this book, we describe the pertinent device technologies and the image quality characteristics of displays used in, or directed at, medical imaging applications.

1.1 Medical Imaging Display Markets

Many medical imaging modalities that rely on display devices for interpretation, review, consultation, or guidance for localization are affected in different ways by the display image quality. This is the case for computed tomography (CT), mammography, chest and bone radiography studies, ultrasound, and image-guided interventional procedures. The assessment of image quality in display devices (both consumer- and medical-grade) has become a key element in the characterization and quality control of diagnostic modalities.

The number of medical imaging procedures performed in the United States is estimated to be about 250 million per year. This figure corresponds to an average of about one procedure per person per year. Using traditional film for display, each procedure is associated with about 3.5 films. The cost of these large-sized films is about $1.60 per sheet, thus indicating a total U.S. market of about $1.4 billion. This estimate is consistent with market estimates made by film manufacturers. Current efforts to replace film with electronic imaging devices are motivated in part by saving the cost of this film, in addition to the overhead associated with film processing and storage.

Each of the estimated 250 million annual medical imaging studies performed in the U.S. needs to be displayed and interpreted by specialists. Most of these specialists are credentialed radiologists. Since the total pool of specialists is about 50,000, these studies are reviewed at the rate of about 25 per day (5,000 per year, 200 days per year). If all studies were to be done on electronic devices, a total of 50,000 workstations would need to be deployed. Additionally, each study may also be reviewed by a referring physician or specialist such as a surgeon. We estimate that this additional review occurs on the average of once per study. For a total pool of 100,000 clinical specialists, this corresponds to 10 reviews of medical displays per day (2500 per year, 250 days) and 100,000 workstations.

If we assume that each of the above 150,000 workstations has two medical monitors each, the total number of monitors deployed in the U.S. would be 300,000. If conversion from film to electronic display occurs within five years for products with a five-year lifetime, this would suggest annual monitor sales of 60,000. The world market for medical imaging equipment is about five times the U.S. market, which would imply an annual world sales market of 300,000 monitors.

While the estimated demand for medical monitors is notable, it should be realized that this market is very small compared to the demand for consumer and business products. As a consequence, the high-performance medical devices that feature controlled gray scale are often dependant on technologies developed for these other larger markets.

Nevertheless, the field of medical displays has experienced considerable growth in recent years. Consider, for instance, the number of display devices offering novel technology in the commercial exhibition of the RSNA Annual Meeting from 1997 to 2002. As presented in Fig. 1.1, devices with new technology are increasingly being demonstrated at the meeting, covering all applications from displays for portable PC's and cellular phones to front-projection devices.

The above-mentioned estimates do not include the myriad of portable devices that are invading the practice of medicine. These devices include "imaging-capable" personal digital assistants,[57] cellular phones, and many varieties of portable computers with a wide range of image quality characteristics. Also missing in the inventory described above are the home computers that are available to radiologists for remote interpretation and consultation. These remote displays typically have a consumer-grade display for which image quality is rarely controlled or assessed.

1.2 Units of Measure

We will use only those units of measure that are required to perform the tests of display image quality described in this book. For more detailed descriptions of photometric and radiometric units, readers are referred to Ref. [32].

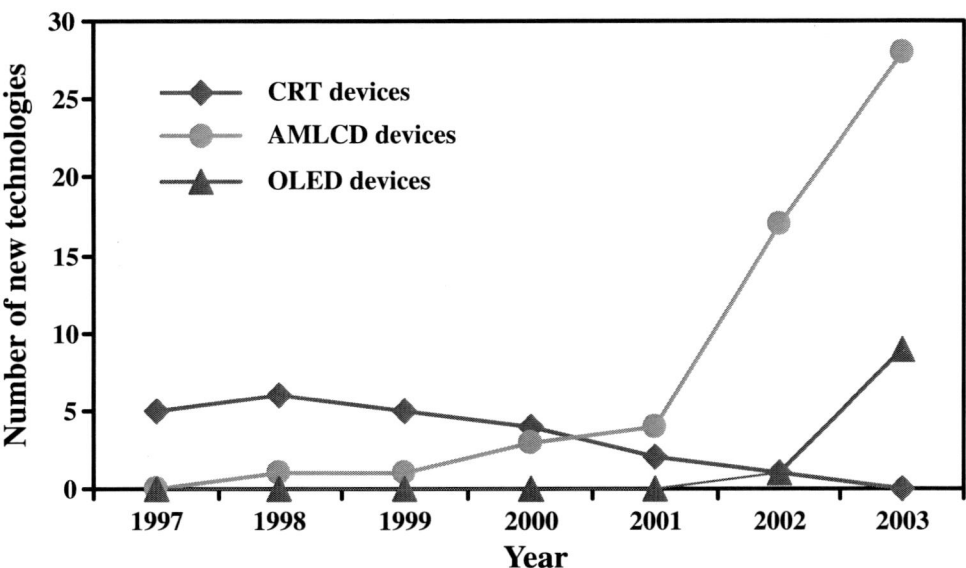

Figure 1.1 Number of display devices offering new technology in the commercial exhibition of the Radiological Society of North America Annual Meeting (1997–2002). The numbers for AMLCDs include gray-scale projection devices. The data were collected by A. Badano from the RSNA's Commercial Exhibit Guide. The 2003 data is a projection by the authors.

We start by introducing the quantities associated with radiometry. Radiometry is the measurement of electromagnetic radiant energy. The most commonly encountered radiometric quantities are listed below:

- Radiant energy: total radiant energy emitted from a emissive source (unit: J)
- Radiant energy density: radiant energy per unit volume (unit: J/m^3)
- Radiant power: flow of radiant energy per unit time (unit: W)
- Radiant intensity: total radiant flux per unit solid angle (unit: W/Sr)
- Irradiance: total radiant flux incident on an element of surface divided by the surface area of the element (unit: W/m^2)
- Radiance: radiant intensity per unit emitting surface area (unit: $W/Sr\cdot m^2$)

Photometry, on the other hand, is the measurement of electromagnetic radiant energy from 380 nm to 760 nm that is sensitive to the human eye. The photometric parameters are radiometric metrics weighted by the eye response of the "standard observer." The eye response of the standard observer is defined by the Commission Internationale de l'Eclairage (CIE). By definition, 1 W in radiometry corresponds to 683 photopic lumens at 555 nm, and 1700 scotopic lumens at 507 nm in photometry. All photometric parameters can be obtained from radiometric quantities by superimposing the CIE photopic sensitivity curve using the following equation:

$$P = 683(\text{lm/W}) \int SR(\lambda)V(\lambda)d\lambda , \qquad (1.1)$$

where P is the photometric parameter (in units of lumen), $SR(\lambda)$ is the spectral radiometric quantity (in units of W), and $V(\lambda)$ is the CIE photopic sensitivity curve.

The basic unit of the photometric parameters is the lumen (lm). The following is the list of photometric parameters and their corresponding units:

- Luminous energy: time integral of luminous flux (unit: lm·sec)
- Luminous energy density: luminous energy per unit volume (unit: lm·sec/m^3)
- Luminous flux: total luminous power emitted from a source (unit: lm)
- Luminous intensity: luminous flux per unit solid angle (unit: lm/Sr or cd)
- Illuminance: density of the luminous flux incident on a surface (unit: lm/m^2 or lux)
- Luminance: ratio of luminous intensity to the area of the source (unit: cd/m^2)

The most important photometric parameters are luminance and illuminance. Luminance is defined as the visible luminous intensity per unit area projected in a given direction. As noted above, the SI unit is the candela per square meter (cd/m^2). The foot-lambert (fL), also in common use, is given by 1 fL = 3.426 cd/m^2. Luminance is often confused with brightness. Brightness is not a physical quantity, and therefore cannot be measured. It is a perceptual quantity attributed to an object by a human. In general, brightness is defined in reference to a well characterized surface or object having high reflectance.

The luminance level of a display or a piece of white paper under room light is typically on the order of 100 cd/m^2. A clear sky in the daylight and a fluorescence lamp have about 3,000 and 5,000–6,000 cd/m^2, respectively. The tolerance limit for human eyes is around 100,000 cd/m^2, and the visible threshold of eyes in darkness is around 0.00001 cd/m^2.

Illuminance is defined as the quantity of visible light striking a surface per unit time. It is associated with the measurement of the brightness of a point source of light as it appears to the eye. It is measured in lux (lm/m^2). The foot-candle is defined as the illuminance on a uniform surface one foot away from the light of one candle and is equal to 1 lm/ft^2. Thus, a light source with an output of 1 lumen flowing through a sphere with a surface area equal to 1 m^2 would produce an illuminance of 1 lux on the surface of the sphere. Conversely, for a light meter to read 1 lux from a uniform point source of light that is 1 m away, a light source of about 12.57 lm is required.

Chapter 2
High-Fidelity Display Performance

All I want to say is that "High Fidelity" has no deep significance.

—Roger Ebert

The purpose of a display device is to convey information to an observer with minimal alteration of its content. All display devices present the information as a modulated luminance map that is associated with the data in the input signal according to a display presentation function. The amount of information detail (i.e., diagnostic information) to be displayed typically determines the quality with which the device must transfer digital values into luminance output. For instance, an alphanumeric device with only seven pixels can display numbers and letters reasonably well on a billboard. When the amount of information to be displayed increases in spatial detail and intensity variations, some degradation in the image quality conveyed to the observer is unavoidable. This is particularly true for some digital medical imaging modalities where large pixel arrays are acquired with a very large image value luminance range.

When electronic displays are used to present large amounts of information (for instance, in digital medical imaging systems for mammography and chest radiography), the image quality requirements are no longer defined by the information content, but instead by the capabilities of the observer to successfully accomplish the visual task. It is therefore essential for those interested in studying the display of high-information content images in electronic devices to understand the observer's limitations. In this chapter, we review aspects of the human visual system relevant to the high-fidelity display requirements of contrast, luminance range, and resolution.

2.1 Contrast Sensitivity

In human vision research, small visual stimuli containing sinusoidal variations in luminance have been used to measure the ability of an observer to perceive contrast. In psychophysics experiments, it is useful to define a measurable quantity, the physical contrast C_{phys}, as

$$C_{phys} = \frac{L_{max} - L_{avg}}{L_{avg}} , \qquad (2.1)$$

where L_{max} is the maximum luminance generated by the display within the pattern and L_{avg} is the mean luminance in the pattern, or mean local luminance.[*] When we refer to mean local luminance, we are assuming that the mean is obtained across the luminance field that contains the pattern or stimulus, as well as some of the background depending on the size of the pattern. However, in this discussion, we will not address the issue of extent of the visual field and its influence on visual detection tasks.

The human eye perceives luminance variations as a change of photoreceptor signal with respect to the viewing angle while scanning a displayed image. It is useful to relate vision data expressed in cycles/degree (cy/deg) to its equivalent in cy/mm at a specified viewing distance VD (mm) using the following expression:

$$cy/mm = 57.3 \ (cy/deg)/VD . \qquad (2.2)$$

For a typical viewing distance of 600 mm, cy/mm is approximately one-tenth of cy/deg.

The minimum contrast detected by the human eye is called the contrast threshold, expressed in relative luminance increment $\Delta L/L$, where L is the local mean luminance. The threshold is also defined as the inverse of the contrast sensitivity response function. The contrast threshold depends on the spatial frequency of the signal and on the relative orientation of the grating to the eye. The threshold also depends on the maximum luminance in the target. The threshold for detection decreases with increasing luminance, as can be seen in Fig. 2.1. The decrease in sensitivity at low luminance is known as the Weber-Fechner law.[149] For a luminance greater than 100 cd/m^2, the threshold is situated at about 0.005. Extensive experimental models have documented the dependence of contrast detection on spatial frequency, luminance, and orientation. The empirical models of Daly[48] and Barten[18, 20] provide useful descriptions of this experimental data.

At high luminance where the threshold contrast $\Delta L/L$ is approximately constant, a gray-scale map for which $\log(L)$ is proportional to the image values will produce uniform contrast. However, for many display systems, the dim regions occur at a luminance where the contrast threshold is high.[135] A gray-scale map can be defined such that each increment in image value causes the same perceived change in luminance.[30] Systems with fewer gray levels may produce noticeable artifacts appearing as contour lines. The low sensitivity of the human visual system

---

[*] Throughout this book, we will use this and other definitions of contrast based on the Michelson contrast.[121] When not specified, the contrast will be given consistently with the above definition, as $\Delta L/L$, where L is the average local luminance.

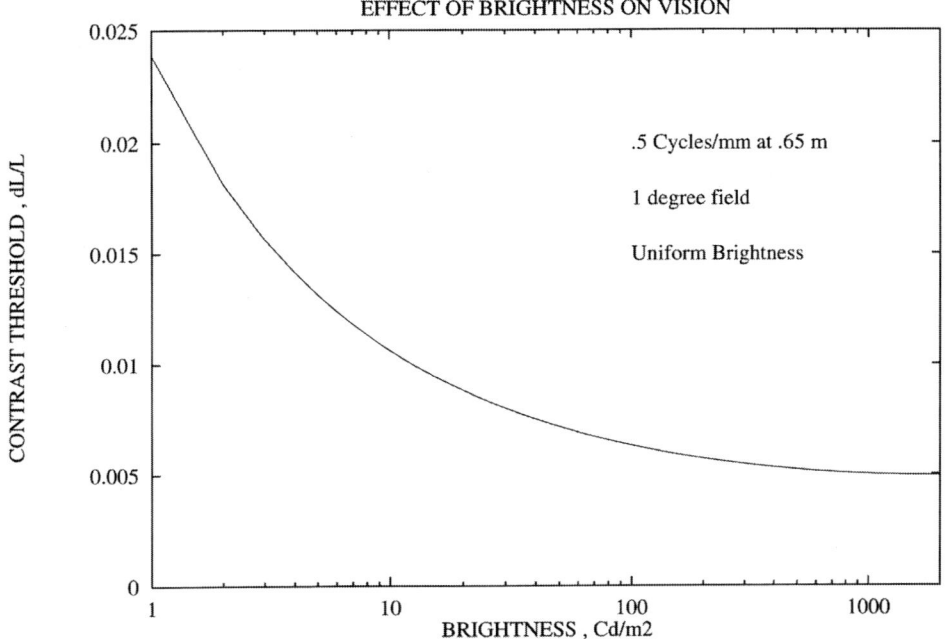

Figure 2.1 Visual contrast threshold as a function of luminance for 0.5 cy/mm at 65 cm. Reproduced with permission from Ref. [137].

to contrast modulation at low luminance is the basis for the perceptually linear display response function discussed in the next section.

2.2 Luminance Response

In the gray-scale display function proposed in the DICOM (Digital Imaging and Communications in Medicine) standard,[2] the contrast in the low luminance region is increased by increasing the slope of the logarithmic representation of luminance against display image values (see Fig. 2.2). For each unit change in the display intensity value, the relative change in luminance $\Delta L/L$ increases the perceived contrast to accommodate sensitivity changes in the human eye.

An important concept that is relevant to human vision systems and displays is the just noticeable difference (JND). The JND, the smallest luminance difference that a human observer can perceive at a given background luminance, is defined as the relative change in luminance equal to the contrast threshold at a given local luminance. In other words, a JND is the increment needed in the image value for the human observer to detect a noticeable change in the display luminance.

The maximum possible number of JNDs associated with a display is determined by the minimum and maximum luminance (L_{min} and L_{max}). For two displays with equal luminance ranges, the one with a higher luminance yields a greater

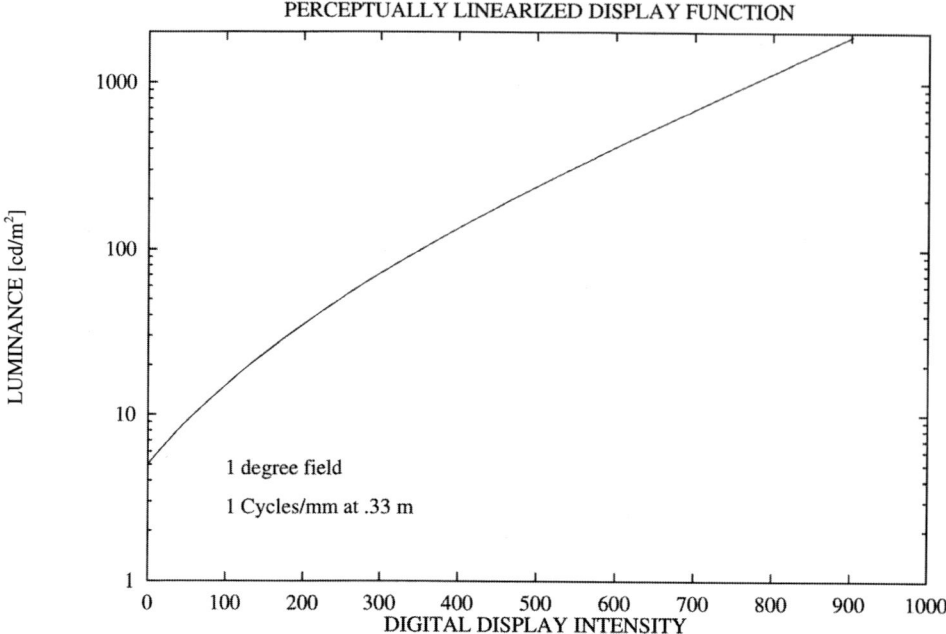

Figure 2.2 A perceptually linear display function. The curve relates the digital display intensity (digital driving level, gray level) to the output luminance as measured in front of the display by some kind of luminance meter (see Sec. 6.1). Equal increments in digital values do not yield equal increments in luminance, but equal increments in perceived contrast. Reproduced with permission from Ref. [137].

number of achievable JNDs. If the same image information is mapped to the less bright display device, the number of available JNDs decreases (see Table 2.1) and the image will be perceived as having lower contrast. Table 2.1 shows the number of achievable JNDs for display devices having different L_{max} levels.

Table 2.1   Number of achievable JNDs for display devices.

L_{max} (cd/m^2)	JNDs
120	450
240	530
480	600
1200	680
2400	730

2.3 Luminance Range

The display luminance range is defined as the ratio of the maximum luminance to the minimum luminance as measured at the screen of the device. Per this definition, the range includes the effect of the ambient illumination as it increases the minimum luminance that the device will output in a dark environment.

The luminance range for which the human eye responds covers eight decades. The neural response of photoreceptors is known to be linear at low light levels and to saturate at high luminance levels.[23, 130] However, in a given scene, the eye adapts to a particular average luminance with a peak response that degrades as the luminance of the target differs more and more from the adapting luminance. Therefore, even though the human visual system is capable of responding to a huge luminance range, the effective range where the eye performs within a fraction of the peak response is limited and depends heavily on the eye's luminance adaptation state.

2.4 Adaptation

The human eye's adaptation to varying luminance levels consists of different phases resulting from the dynamics of the chemicals responsible for vision.[79, 80, 129] Using electrophysiological observations and computer simulations, Norman[128] and Baxter[22] reported on the relationship between photoreceptor sensitivity and image processing at neural centers for visual tasks involving the detection of low-contrast radiological features in nonuniform backgrounds. The sensitivity response function for the complete visual system can be approximately described by an expression of the form $P = R/(R + S)$, where P is the photoreceptor response, R is the retinal luminous intensity, and S represents a constant that conforms with the state of adaptation. Figure 2.3 shows the measured neuronal signal for different adaptation states.

When the observer is adapted to a particular average luminance, the perceived contrast response is maximal near the average luminance and decreases in regions of the scene with higher or lower luminance, as shown in Fig. 2.4. Displaying images using a wide luminance range improves quality due to the high physical contrast (large $\Delta L/L$ for a specific image intensity change). However, the perceived contrast is a combination of the physical contrast and the observer's biological response. Therefore, for a typical scene with luminance variations about a scene average, contrast perception is reduced in the bright and dim areas relative to the maximum performance at the average luminance for which the eye is adapted.

The question arises as to what might be the optimal adaptation luminance (other than the display device). The above-mentioned arguments suggest that for slowly variant luminance fields, the average luminance has to be close to the average image luminance. This observation—that the optimal background luminance for human visual detection tasks has to be close to the average luminance of the observed scene—is opposed to conventional reading conditions with extremely low

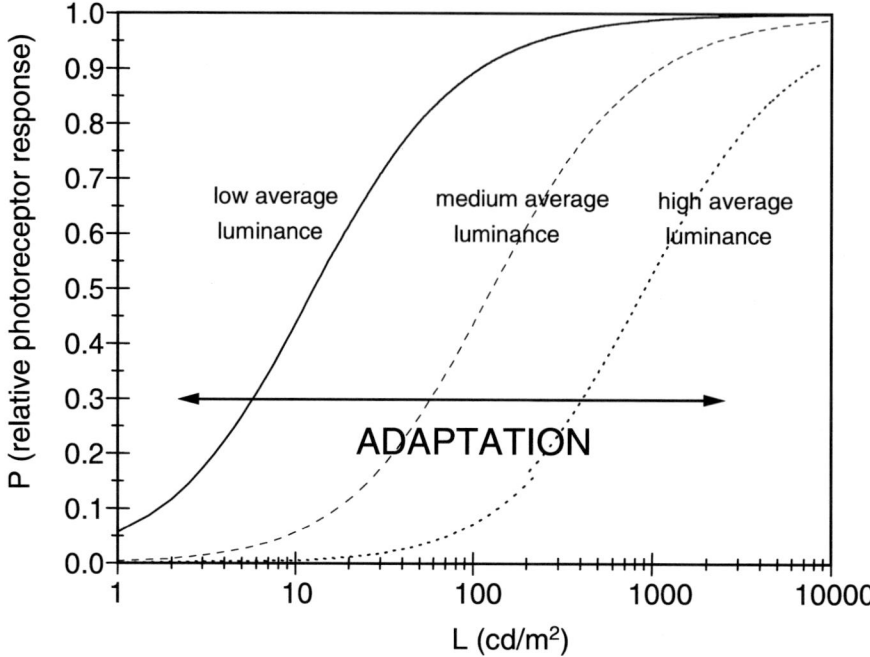

Figure 2.3 Adaptation of the photoreceptors to low, medium, and high average scene luminance. Reproduced from Ref. [61] with permission of the RSNA.

ambient illuminance. The luminance of areas surrounding an image should then be similar to the average image luminance. In addition, spatial equalization by digital image processing helps maintain contrast in all areas of a scene. From Fig. 2.4, we conclude that human vision can perceive contrast over an average luminance range of about 80 in order for the adapted visual system to maintain satisfactory contrast response (i.e., in excess of 35% of the maximum response). The overall size of the field that contributes to adaptation is probably about 100 mm (500 mm viewing distance) in diameter. To permit objects with a contrast of 1.0 in dark regions (at L_{min}) and in bright regions (at L_{max}), the minimum luminance should be 0.5 and the maximum 120, resulting in a full luminance range of 240. This corresponds to a film density (i.e., optical density) range of 2.4.

2.5 Retinal Anatomy and Visual Acuity

The resolution limit of the human eye is determined mostly by the distribution of photoreceptors in the eye's retina. The retina is a complex multilayer lining of the posterior inner surface of the eyeball. In addition to the light-sensitive cells, the retina is formed by a set of networked nerve cells responsible for the transmission (and initial processing stages) of the signals. Two main classes of photoreceptors can be found in the retina: cones and rods. Cone receptors are highly concentrated

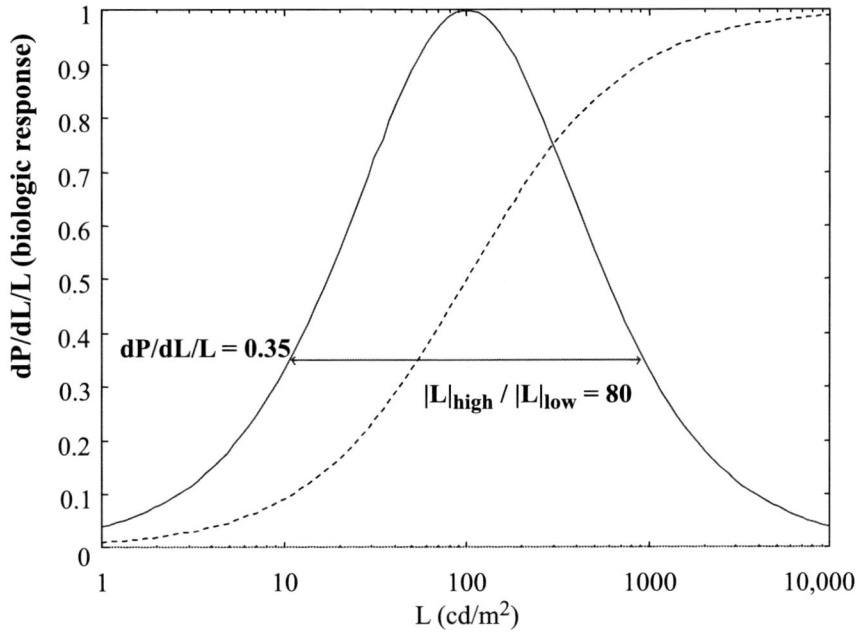

Figure 2.4 Luminance range for good contrast response. Using one of the adaptation curves presented in Fig. 2.3 (dashed curve), we can compute the contrast response profiles (solid curve) for that particular adaptation state. The profiles, which exhibit a peak at the inflexion point of the luminance response curves, describe how the observer's contrast response performance is only maximum at one particular luminance level (100 cd/m²) while being lower for any other luminance. The luminance range of 80 indicated in the figure defines a luminance range for which the contrast response is 0.35 of the maximum or higher. Adapted from Ref. [61] with permission of the RSNA.

in a small region called the fovea. The high density of photoreceptors in the fovea results in high acuity. In addition, three types of cones are responsible for color vision due to their differing sensitivity across the visible spectrum:

1. S-cones (blue), with peak sensitivity at 437 nm, constituting about 2 % of the total number of cones;

2. M-cones (green), with peak sensitivity at 533 nm, constituting about 33 % of the total number of cones; and

3. L-cones (red), with peak sensitivity at 564 nm, constituting about 65 % of the total number of cones.

   Rods populate the more peripheral areas of the retina with a maximum density at about 20–30 deg from the fovea. The lower density of photoreceptors in the periphery produces lower acuity in that region of the retina. However, rods are more sensitive to light, and are therefore used mostly for night or low-light vision.

   The resolving power of the human visual system depends strongly on the frequency of the target. This can be seen in Fig. 2.5 expressed at a viewing distance

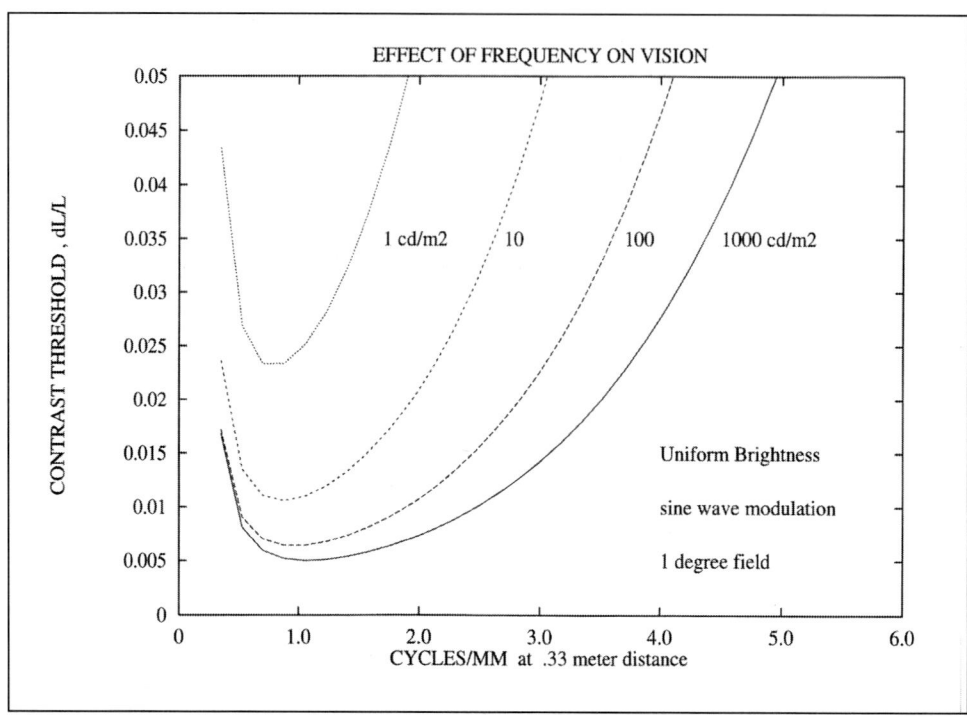

Figure 2.5 Effect of the spatial frequency of the stimulus on vision threshold. Reproduced with permission from Ref. [62].

of 33 cm. Figure 2.5 shows how the contrast threshold varies with the spatial frequency of the stimulus. The spatial frequency for the minimum threshold for each of the curves presented occurs at about the same frequency (close to 1 cy/mm). For a higher luminance, the frequency of the minimum threshold increases slightly. We also note that the magnitude of the threshold changes with luminance, as discussed in previous sections.

The pixel size of a display system that matches the resolving power of the human eye depends on the observation distance and on the display luminance. For a square wave pattern with a contrast of 0.05, the maximum cy/mm and minimum pixel size are given in Table 2.2.

Table 2.2 Pixel sizes corresponding to maximum spatial acuity of the human visual system.

Viewing Distance	$L_{max} = 100$ cd/m^2	$L_{max} = 1,000$ cd/m^2
At close inspection (33 m)	4 cy/mm 0.125 mm/pixel	5 cy/mm 0.100 mm/pixel
At normal viewing (66 m)	2 cy/mm 0.250 mm/pixel	2.5 cy/mm 0.200 mm/pixel

2.6 Veiling Glare

In this section, we will discuss two aspects of veiling glare: first, we will consider how veiling glare in the human eye affects detection tasks, and second, we will describe the intrinsic veiling glare characteristics of displays. Both aspects relate to the same physical phenomenon: the undesired degradation in display contrast caused by unwanted scattering processes. In the case of the human eye, veiling glare is caused primarily by optical scattering of light in the anatomical elements through which the light traverses before reaching the photoreceptors in the retina. In displays, the causes of glare are associated with optical and/or electronic scattering. Information about measuring veiling glare in displays is covered in Sec. 6.2.1.

2.6.1 Glare in the human eye

The human eye is able to discriminate the orientation of light photons that enter the eye due to its sharp angular sensitivity response to light that impinges into the retina at oblique angles (see Fig. 2.6). Light that originates at the focused object, which is responsible for the viewed image, is scattered while passing through several media, including the cornea, the aqueous humor, and the crystalline lens. Because of this optical scattering process, even a collimated beam of light coming from an external point source will produce an optical illumination in the retina characterized by a blur, or spread function. That spread of signal, equivalent to the point-spread function of the eye,[*] has been studied by many investigators.[25] A good review of glare processes in the human eye can be found in Ref. [152]. In that paper, Spencer et al. classified glare effects into two components: flare and bloom. Flare, seen as a halo, is caused primarily by scattering events in the lens, while blooming (or "glowing") comes from events in the lens, the retina, and the cornea. The retinal scattering is important only in the same direction as the incident primary beam due to the extremely low sensitivity of the cones to obliquely incident rays (known as the Crawford-Stiles effect[153, 154]). In scotopic conditions (low luminance levels), the magnitude of glare in the eye increases because the rods do not have as high a directional sensitivity as the cones. Although lacking specific quantitative value, the point-spread function of the human eye has been represented in many artistic pieces, including that of Fig. 2.7. Veiling glare in the human eye is not believed to have an effect on typical reading conditions since the luminance of radiologic images consists of small variations about a scene average in an environment with overall low ambient illuminance. On the other hand, veiling glare does affect image quality in some display technologies.

---

[*] The point-spread function is defined here as a general response function in the human eye caused by a small light source far away from the receptor, emitting light photons into a collimated pencil beam.

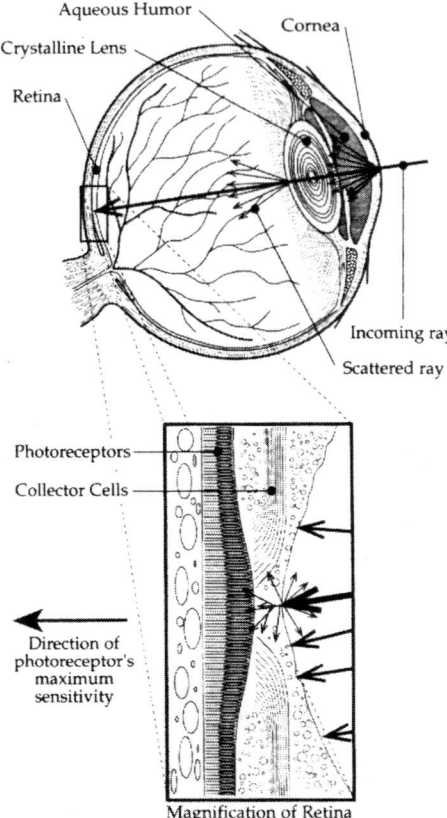

Figure 2.6 The scattering of a beam of light entering the eye with events in the lens, cornea, and retina. Reprinted from Ref. [152] with permission of the IEEE.

2.6.2 Veiling glare in displays

Veiling glare in display devices represents a significant source of image quality degradation. Particularly for medical CRT monitors, manufacturers have developed solutions to control veiling glare. Although a different phenomenon seen in high-resolution AMLCDs known as electronic crosstalk also reduces display contrast, it is not characterized as veiling glare because of its distinct origins. Electronic crosstalk is discussed in detail in Sec. 4.5.

2.6.2.1 Sources of glare

Veiling glare in displays is commonly associated with the multiple light-scattering processes that take place in the emissive structures of a CRT, causing a contrast reduction that is most significant in low-luminance regions surrounded by bright

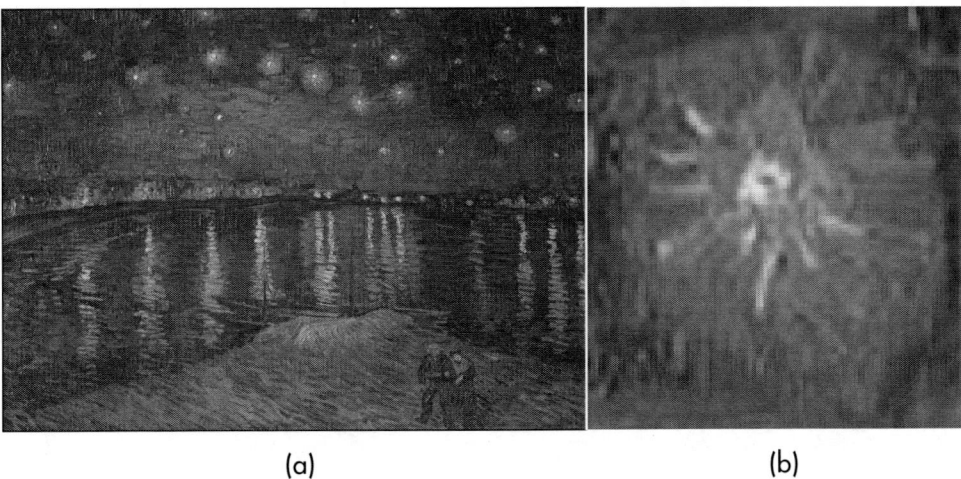

(a)   (b)

Figure 2.7   Veiling glare in the human eye. (a) Reproduction of the painting by Vincent van Gogh, *La nuit étoilée (Starry Night over the Rhône)*, 1888 (RF 1975–19), Paris, Musée d'Orsay, donation de M. et Mme. Robert Kahn-Sriber, 1975. In his representations of stars, van Gogh portrays the spread of signal in the human visual system. In (b), one illustration of a star is enlarged to appreciate the details. Reproduced with permission of the Musée d'Orsay.

areas (see Fig. 2.8). Although veiling glare is typically associated with optical scattering or light diffusion, other sources of veiling glare (such as light leakage and electron backscattering) are less known, but also merit a detailed description (see Fig. 2.9).

Light diffusion. To reduce veiling glare, high-performance monochrome and color CRTs typically have an absorptive face plate that reduces the brightness. Other approaches that have been implemented in color designs include filtered and pigmented phosphor grains.[95] All color tubes presently have a black absorptive matrix between phosphor dots that improves the display contrast as well as the achievable color purity, which results in a larger color gamut. The absorption of light by this layer greatly reduces the magnitude of the tails of the spread functions associated with veiling glare.[4] The contribution of veiling glare due to light transport processes within the emissive structure depends proportionally on the relative location of dark and bright regions in an image. Therefore, its effect is determined by the spatial luminance distribution of each image scene. Conversely, the other two mechanisms that contribute to glare, which will be analyzed next, cause a background signal that is approximately uniform throughout the entire display surface.

Light leakage. The reflectivity of Al-backed films used in CRTs is typically on the order of 90% or greater. The transmitted light scatters off the walls of the bulb and may eventually exit through the face plate, adding a uniform undesired background to the image. This light leakage has been recognized and used as part of an experimental method to determine the Al layer thickness,[54] and for adjusting the display

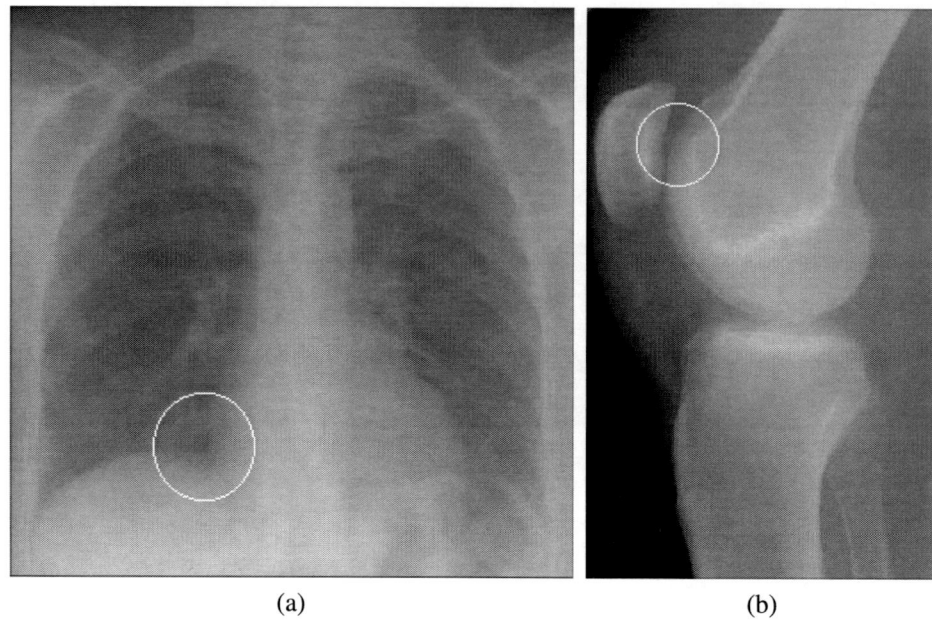

(a)   (b)

Figure 2.8 Radiographic images showing significant veiling glare effects. White circles indicate regions where the conspicuity of subtle detail in dark regions is affected by veiling glare from the bright surroundings.

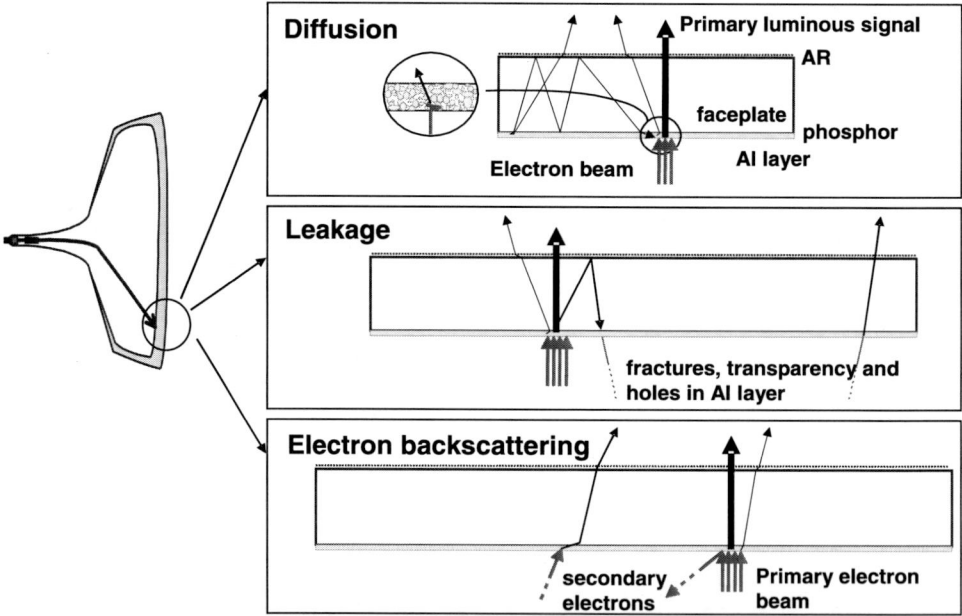

Figure 2.9 Schematic representation of the three sources of veiling glare: light diffusion, light leakage, and electron backscattering. Reproduced from Ref. [6] with permission of the RSNA.

curve according to illuminance measurements made inside the CRT bulb. When the transmitted light intensity through the Al film amounts to 10%, a uniform bright field will be contaminated by an additional constant luminance of 5×10^{-4} times the bright field intensity. This figure assumes 90% absorption of all scattering events at the walls of the tube. Typically, coatings for the inside surfaces of CRT bulbs are carbon-based absorptive materials, although metallic coatings containing Cu and Ag are also used in certain applications. If a small dark spot is placed in the center of an image at a luminance level of 1% of the bright field, its physical contrast will decrease from 99 to 94. In addition, the thin Al coating that covers the phosphor layer may have small cracks or holes that will allow more light generated in the phosphor to escape towards the vacuum cell, resulting in a further decrease in contrast.

Electron backscattering. In addition to an optical component, a significant contribution of glare in displays is caused by electron backscattering. The reduction in contrast due to backscattered electrons has been studied for fluorescent screens[114] and for scanning electron microscopes.[74] To obtain good color saturation, a shadow mask is located in front of the screen to allow each electron beam to selectively pass through the mask holes and excite the corresponding color phosphor. Although the beams are focused and aligned with the holes, a fraction of the Gaussian-shaped beam will directly hit the mask. As some energetic electrons impinge into the shadow mask or the screen, a fraction is backscattered and may eventually hit the phosphor layer at a different location. Short-range contrast degradation is originated by electron scattering in the vacuum region between the mask and the phosphor screen, while the long-range effect comes from backscattering at the mask and at the inner magnetic shield and funnel of the glass bulb.[52] The aperture grille used with in-line electron guns, introduced in 1988, represents another approach employed for color selection. The transmittance of the beam is 15 to 50% greater compared to shadow mask designs.

The backscattered fraction depends on the effective atomic number of the coating, and therefore can be reduced by using low-Z materials such as graphite[161] or Al_2O_3.[162] The amount of contrast reduction from backscattering is directly proportional to the primary beam intensity. It has been reported that the fraction of contrast loss due to electronic backscattering in color tubes can be as much as 98% of the total glare degradation.[52] Reduction by a factor of about 10 in the contrast ratio of 10×10 cm black squares can be achieved by careful selection of coating material and thickness. The absence of a shadow mask in monochrome tubes results in a lower backscattered fraction since all the electrons hit the Al conductive coating and phosphor layer.

2.6.2.2 Effect of veiling glare

The human visual system is able to detect a dark region having less than 0.002 of the luminance of a bright surrounding field. We can conclude that a display device should not add significant luminance to dark regions surrounded by bright fields. It

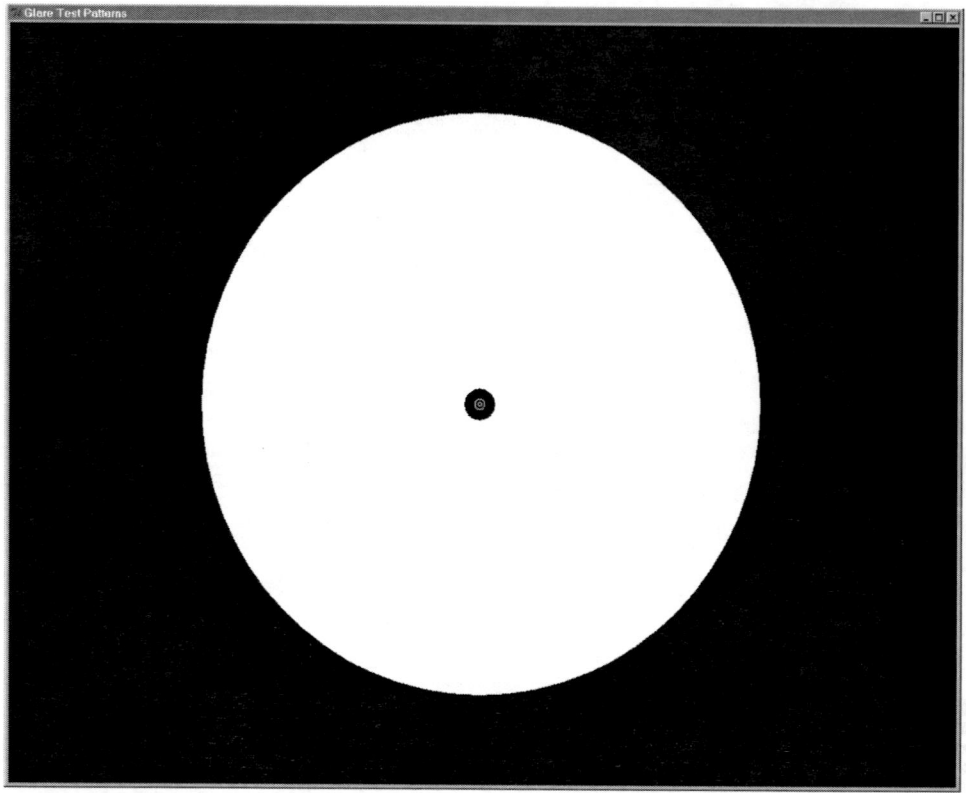

Figure 2.10   Image test pattern to illustrate and measure veiling glare effects.

is useful to define a veiling glare ratio (G) as the ratio of the luminance of the bright surroundings to the luminance of a small dark spot [see Eq. (6.2)]. Using this ratio, which can be measured experimentally (see Fig. 2.10), we can determine the requirements for a high-fidelity display device. If the luminance change in dark areas due to veiling glare should be less than 20% with an average luminance range of 80, the contribution from glare in the dark regions should be less than 0.20. Thus, the required glare ratio in this condition is $G = 80/0.20 = 400$.

2.7 Ambient Light Reflections

In this section, we will discuss how the performance of a human observer is critically affected by the level and nature of the ambient illumination. As can be seen in Fig. 2.11, the displayed image can be buried under high reflected luminance. Particularly for CRT devices, reflections can be represented by the addition of a specular and a diffuse component (see Figs. 2.12 and 2.13) with different effects on the quality of the image displayed. More generally, reflections include a third component called "haze," which becomes important in flat-panel LCDs (see Chapter 4).

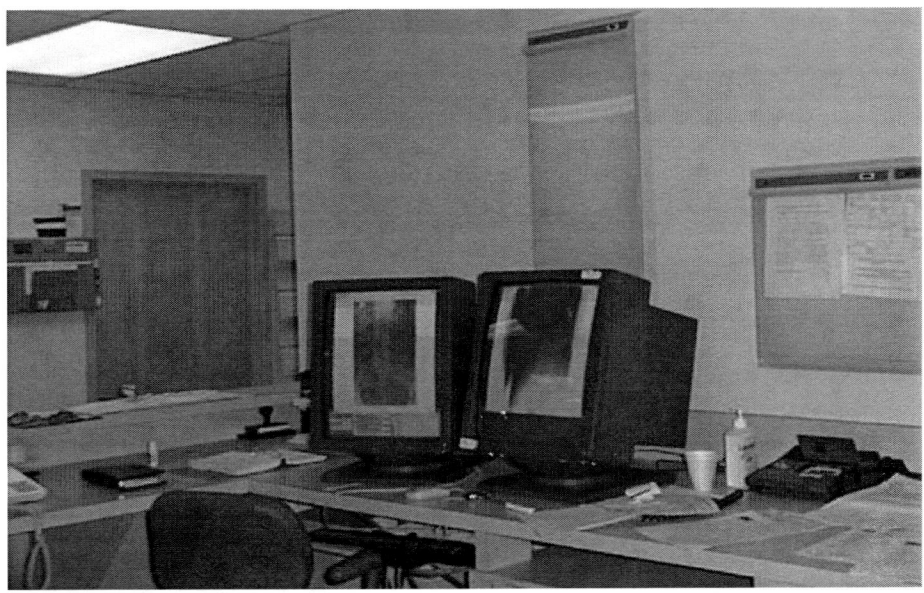

Figure 2.11 Typical radiological workstation with poor room illumination control.

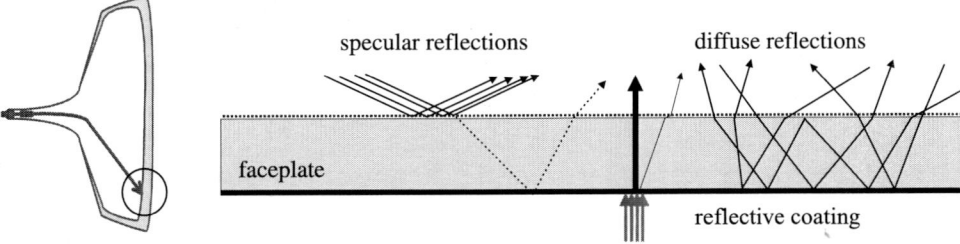

Figure 2.12 Specular and diffuse reflections for a CRT. The solid lines indicate the position of the electron beam and the luminance that it generates upon impinging into the phosphor layer. The specular reflections occur mostly at the front surface of the face plate. The dotted line represents a specular reflection at the back surface. The reflective coating, designed primarily to increase the light output of the phosphor, also increases the diffuse component of the display reflections. Reproduced from Ref. [6] with permission of the RSNA.

2.7.1 Specular reflection

The brightness of a white object (with 90% diffuse reflectivity) illuminated by I lux is given by $0.9I/\pi$ cd/m^2. In this case, we can establish that the change in luminance caused by the reflection of that white object should be below the visible contrast threshold (C_t) at the minimum luminance (L_{min}) defined as $C_t = \Delta L/L_{min}$, where L_{min} is the display luminance at the minimum of its luminance response.

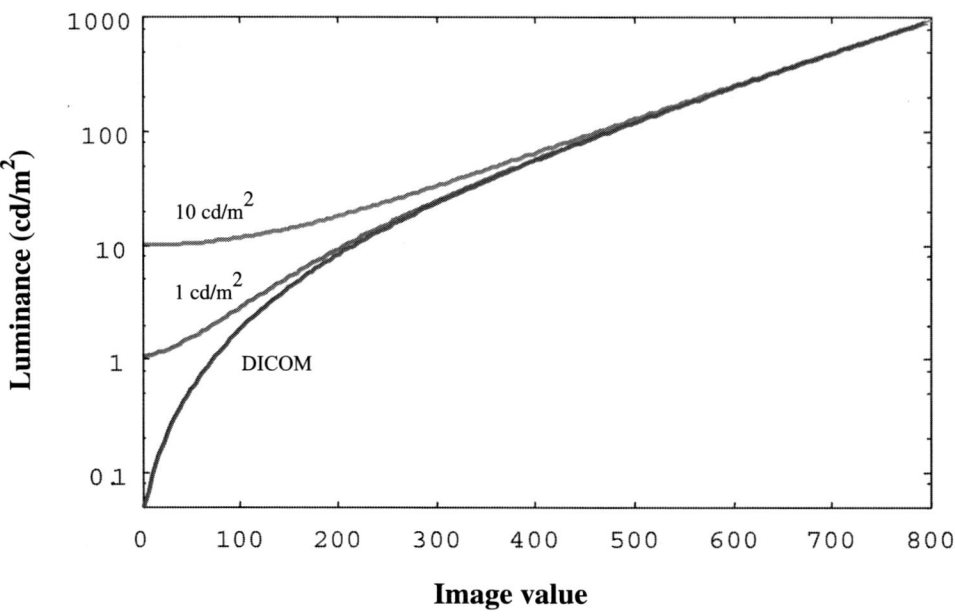

Figure 2.13 Contrast reduction from diffuse added luminance. The slope of the gray-scale display function is directly related to the contrast of the display at a given luminance level. Increasing ambient illumination to 1 and 10 cd/m² leads to a reduction in the available contrast in the low luminance regions.

For instance, the contrast threshold at 4 cd/m² is 0.012 (see Fig. 2.1). In a room with an illumination of 100 lux at the display screen, the reflected specular luminance is given by $0.9 \times 100/\pi$ (cd/m²). This reflected luminance should be less than the threshold luminance at 4 cd/m², given by 4×0.012 cd/m². The specular reflection coefficient, R_S, that satisfies this condition is 0.002. Using this criterion, we can calculate the maximum ambient illumination (in lux) that maintains the specular reflections of white and black objects below C_t. Table 2.3 shows the values calculated for specific display luminance minima. Typical levels of ambient illumination in areas where image displays are found are presented in Table 2.4.

Table 2.3 Ambient illumination (in lux) required for maintaining specular reflections.

L_{min} (cd/m²)	C_t	R_S				
		0.002	0.004	0.008	0.020	0.040
20	0.007	244	122	61	24	12
10	0.008	140	70	35	14	7
4	0.012	84	42	21	8	4
2	0.017	59	30	15	6	3
1	0.024	42	21	10	4	2

Table 2.4 Typical ambient illumination levels.

Space	I (lux)
Operating rooms	300–400
Emergency rooms	150–300
Staff offices	50–180
Clinical viewing areas	200–250
Diagnostic viewing (CT or MR)	15–60
Diagnostic viewing (x ray)	2–10

2.7.2 Diffuse reflection

The diffuse reflection of light adds an unstructured constant luminance to the image that reduces the contrast in dark regions. The diffuse reflection coefficient describes the added luminance per unit illuminance, R_D (cd/m^2/lux). Therefore, the added luminance is given by

$$\Delta L = R_D I . \tag{2.3}$$

To limit the contrast reduction, the relative change in contrast produced by ambient illumination should not be less than 0.8:

$$\frac{1}{(1 + \Delta L/L_{min})} \le 0.8 . \tag{2.4}$$

Using Eq. (2.4), we can calculate the minimum reflection coefficient that will result in a given added luminance for a given room illumination in the front of the screen (illumination is defined as the amount of light impinging into the screen from the ambient and should be measured in the center of the screen). For example, for a display with 4 cd/m^2 of minimum luminance in a room with 100 lux ($I/L_{min} = 25$), the diffuse reflection coefficient is given by

$$R_D \le \frac{1/0.8 - 1}{25} , \tag{2.5}$$

yielding a required R_D of less than 0.01 cd/m^2/lux. The values of room illumination that satisfy this condition are shown in Table 2.5.

Table 2.5   Ambient illumination (in lux) for maintaining 80% of the available contrast in dark regions.

L_{min} (cd/m^2)	R_D (cd/m^2/lux)				
	0.002	0.004	0.008	0.020	0.040
20	1000	500	250	125	83
10	500	250	125	62	42
4	200	100	50	25	17
2	100	50	25	12	8
1	50	25	12	6	4

2.8 High-Fidelity Display Requirements

For the purpose of display requirements, medical tasks can be classified into these two categories:

- **High fidelity (diagnostic).** Primary medical interpretations performed by persons qualified to read radiologic studies. Medical review of radiographs by specialists who have skills in reading studies for a particular purpose (orthopedists, rheumatologists, neurologists, surgeons).

- **Good (clinical).** Preliminary interpretations in urgent care situations. Referring physician observation in conjunction with interpretative reports. Clinical management functions requiring basic anatomic observations (fractures, opaque objects).

As we discussed at the beginning of this chapter, display requirements are strongly dependent on the specific visual task that the observer will carry out. Therefore, a general list of display requirements for radiology is not feasible. Nevertheless, our analysis provides a way to define requirements for high-fidelity display based on the limitations of the human visual system.

Table 2.6 is a summary chart presenting ranges of values for the most relevant display parameters. Details of the method to determine these requirements for most of the parameters listed in the table will be discussed in this book. Other parameters such as area distortion and viewing angle are not based on material from this chapter. Instead, we have included them in this listing for completeness, and they should be taken as suggestions coming from our experience with film display. It should be noted that more research is needed in some of these areas in order to ascertain more precisely the high-fidelity requirements for an electronic display.

Another point to note about these values is that they represent general high-fidelity medical display requirements instead of requirements valid for any given applications. When specific applications are considered, these values will need to

Table 2.6 Display requirements for medical imaging applications.

Specification	Film Quality	High Fidelity	Good Quality
Spatial			
Size (cm)	35 × 43	30 × 36	24 × 30
Pixel array	4000 × 5000	2500 × 3000	1200 × 1500
Pixel size (mm)	0.08	0.12	0.20
Refresh rate (Hz)	static	static – 80	static – 80
Geometrical distortion (%)	< 0.1	2	2
Gray scale			
Maximum luminance (cd/m^2)	2000	1000	240
Minimum luminance (cd/m^2)	1	4	1
Gray-scale levels	> 850	> 680	> 530
Emission	Lambertian	Lambertian	Lambertian
Color	monochrome	monochrome	monochrome
Optical			
Veiling glare ratio	> 1000	400	150
Specular reflectance	0.02	0.002	0.004
Diffuse reflectance (cd/m^2/lux)	0.02	0.01	0.02
Viewing angle (V)	full	± 45°	± 30°
Viewing angle (H)	full	± 60°	± 45°

be adjusted. For instance, it is known that in some diagnostic modalities like mammography and skeletal radiography, the image features that need to be detected for an accurate diagnosis are small. This need forces a more stringent requirement on the display's resolution. On the other hand, when the lesions to be detected are low-contrast, subtle variations in the luminance, a precise luminance calibration and appropriate luminance range might be more important.

Some definitions used in the development of Table 2.6 require additional explanation. The display size of 43 × 35 cm is standard for radiographic detectors. Displays should have a horizontal/vertical aspect ratio of about 0.8. We assume that the log-luminance versus pixel value relationships should follow a perceptually linear profile based on the DICOM standard. With respect to display color, general preference in the field has been for displays with a white to slightly blue color. Most film bases are tinted blue. The contrast ratio for veiling glare measurement is defined with test pattern images consisting of a 1-cm, centered, dark circular spot surrounded by a bright field. With respect to the viewing angle performance, we require that the stated contrast and luminance performances are to be maintained within the required viewing angle, and no contrast inversion is allowed.

Chapter 3
Cathode-Ray Tubes

About thirty-six years ago, a stone of this type was found in the countryside near Bologna by an honest man of humble circumstances who was given the assiduous pursuit of activity in the science of chemistry; he was called Vincenzo Casciarolo, and he was of Bolognian origin. ...After submitting the stone to much preparation, it was not the Pluto of Aristophanes that resulted; instead, it was the Luciferous Stone, which would not itself produce gold, but which would absorb the golden light of the sun, like a new Prometheus stealing a Celestial Treasure.

—Professor Fortunius Licetus, in an excerpt from
Litheosphorus, sive de lapide Bononiensi (1640)

Cathode-ray tube (CRT) technology has been maturing for many decades, from the 1602 discovery of luminescent materials called "phosphors" by Vincenzo Casciarolo, an Italian shoemaker and alchemist, up to the recent development of complex electron optics to control the beam spot impinging into the monitor screen. In 1890, W. Crookes used a CRT for electron shadowing of metallic objects. In 1895, W. K. Roentgen used a tube with similar design as an x-ray generator. An important milestone in the history of the CRT was the tube designed by K. Braun. The "Braun" tube had most of the key elements of current CRTs: an electron source or cathode, a focusing and deflection device, a screen, and a housing. The first commercial CRTs were produced by Western Electric in the early 1920s, but it was not until the 1940s that massive amounts of units were available as consumer products.[96] Current CRT designs provide high image quality for a variety of applications.

In this chapter, we describe the basic elements of a CRT monitor, then explain how color CRT monitors differ from monochrome CRTs with respect to the display image quality. Finally, we describe the characteristics of medical monochrome CRTs used in diagnostic workstations.

The CRT is a cathodo-luminescent display. An electron gun emits an energetic beam that strikes a phosphor screen within a small spot. Magnetic deflection coils steer the beam in a raster scan. Finally, a cathodo-luminescent phosphor con-

25

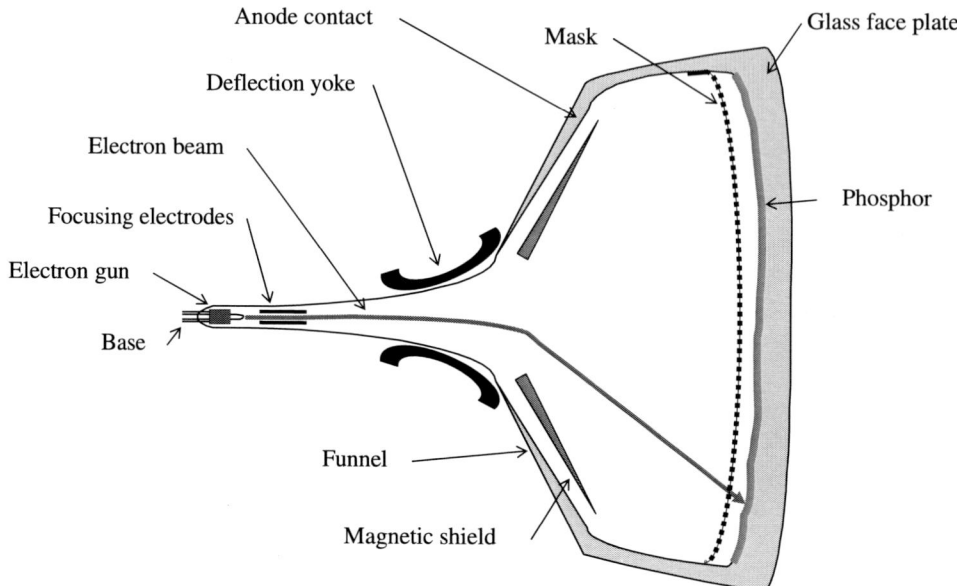

Figure 3.1   The major components of a CRT.

verts electron energy into light. The beam current is modulated to cause varying brightness. Figure 3.1 shows the arrangement of these typical CRT elements. The vacuum inside the large CRT bulb is contained using a thick glass in the funnel and face plate to reduce the mechanical stress. A 74-cm diagonal bulb with a relatively flat face plate requires a glass thickness of about 13 mm.

3.1 Cathodes

In a cathode, electrons are extracted by a resistive heater that promotes thermal emission with temperatures of about 600°C. Two types of cathodes are used in CRTs. In oxide cathodes (Ba, Sr, and Ca oxides), low surface-potential materials are used with an average energy required to extract an electron, W, of less than 1.7 eV at a temperature of 750°C. Oxide cathodes require a continuous vacuum environment. A second type of cathode used in CRTs is the dispenser or impregnated cathode. Dispenser cathodes consist of a porous tungsten (W) pellet impregnated with emissive oxide material. They can achieve a high current density, with a longer lifetime and better stability than oxide cathodes due to the oxide cathode's need for replenishment of oxide material. In addition, dispenser cathodes have excellent aging characteristics, suffering from only about 1% loss in emission for every 1,000 hours (see Fig. 3.2). Degradation in thermionic cathodes occurs due to high-temperature vacuum erosion. Figure 3.3 shows drawings of the two types of cathodes used in high-performance CRTs.

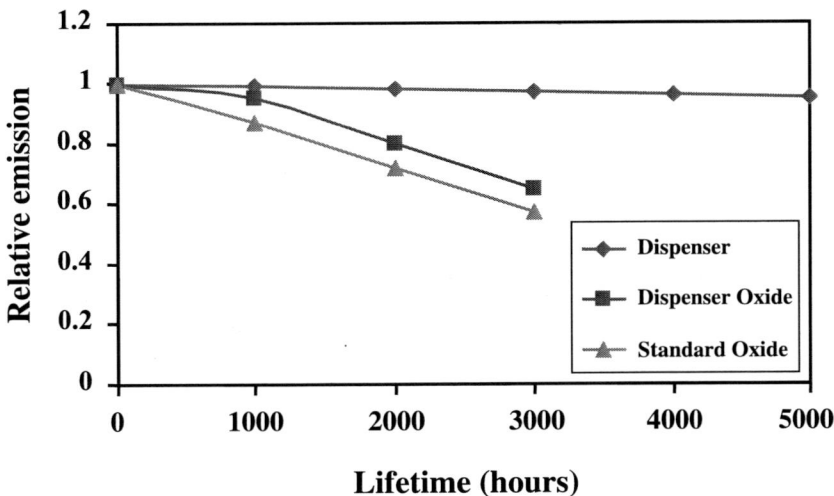

Figure 3.2 Comparison of the reduction in electron emission due to aging of CRT cathodes. The data represent a high-cathode loading with an intensity of 0.4 mA.

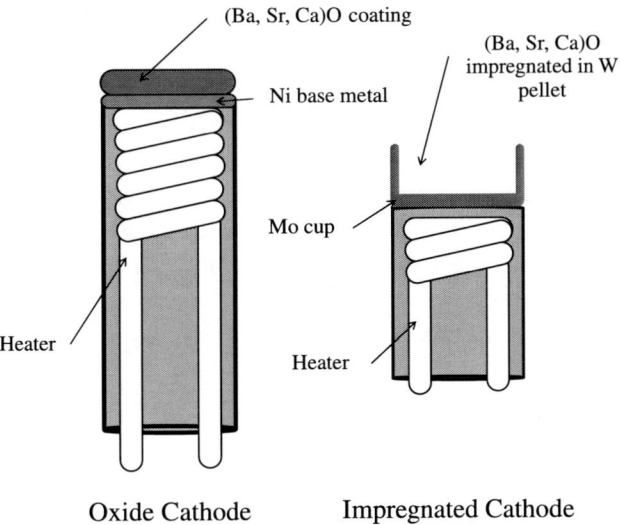

Figure 3.3 Oxide and dispenser thermionic cathodes found in high-performance CRTs.

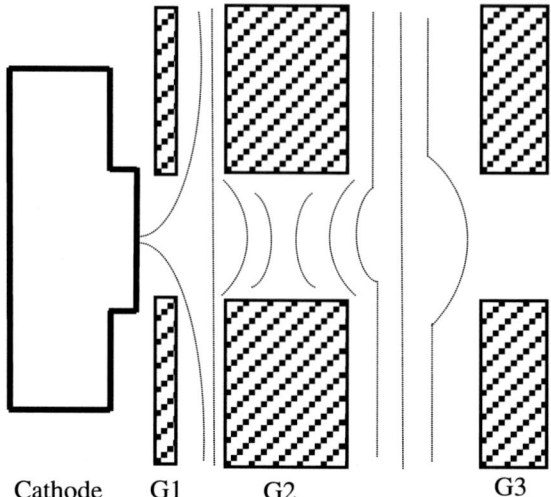

| Cathode | G1 | G2 | G3 |

Figure 3.4 Einzel lens arrangement used in the CRT electron gun. The potential G1 defines the area for the extraction of electrons from the heated cathode. The electron beam is then focused and accelerated through the rest of the lens using potentials G2 and G3.

3.2 Electron Optics

The electron beam generated at the cathode is accelerated and focused by a series of electrostatic lenses that form the electron gun. The Einzel-type lenses have a number of key potentials that shape the beam (see Fig. 3.4). The potential difference between the cathode and the G1 potential defines the emissive area on the cathode surface. The G1, G2, and G3 potentials establish the electric field that focuses the beam.

The electron beam needs to be directed at a particular spot in the emissive screen, which is accomplished by a deflection yoke situated at the exit of the electron gun. The yoke is an external device that is designed to closely fit the shape of the glass bulb. It generates magnetic fields responsible for the beam deflection. The electron beam traverses the majority of the field-free vacuum space until it hits the front screen. The beam's raster pattern causes large angle deflections. In demanding applications where a large screen size with constant image quality across the viewable area is desired, special high-performance yoke designs with dynamic fine control over deflection and focusing are used.

3.3 Emissive Structure

A key component of the CRT that greatly affects its image quality is the emissive structure, consisting of all those elements responsible for the generation and delivery of light—the final step for the presentation of images to the observer. Emissive structures vary greatly according to the type of CRT. In general, they consist of a

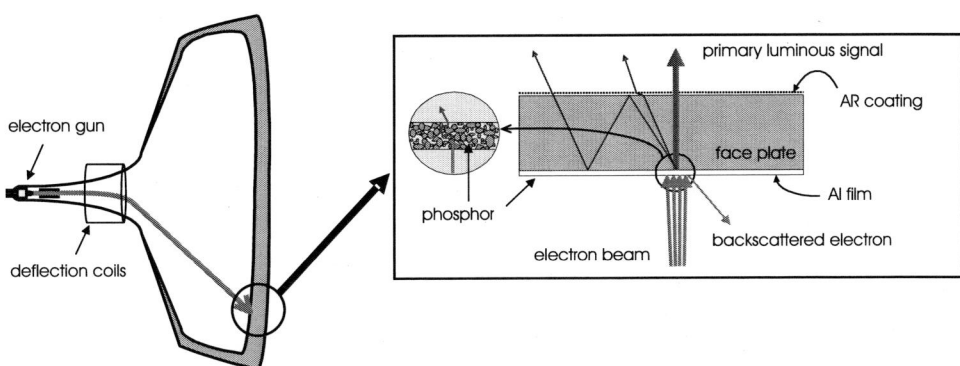

Figure 3.5 Emissive structure of a CRT showing the components where light is generated and conveyed outside of the display device for the observer.

conductive coating (normally a thin Al overcoat), a luminescent phosphor, a black matrix layer, a glass face plate, and sometimes an antireflective coating (see Fig. 3.5). All of these components are described in detail in the following sections, where we address specific CRT designs.

A typical structure consists of a cathodo-luminescent[134] phosphor deposited onto a glass face-plate panel as a powder layer using a sedimentation technique. In color tubes, an absorptive carbon-based black layer known as the "black matrix" separates the RGB phosphor dots for luminance and chromatic contrast. A sub-micron reflective layer of Al is overlaid on top of the phosphor to conduct the incoming electron current and maximize light output towards the viewer. For that purpose, a filming material is used to assure a smooth, continuous, and highly reflective film. Figure 3.6(a) shows a scanning electron microscope image of the emissive structure of a monochrome CRT. Multiple layers of phosphor grains can be observed under the thin Al coating. The glass face-plate can absorb up to 70% of the direct light, thus improving contrast, and may have a rough surface on the vacuum side to reduce specular reflections. A photograph of the interior surface of a CRT face-plate sample after the Al and phosphor layers were removed is shown in Fig. 3.6(b).

3.4 Signal Electronics

The incoming electronic signal in a CRT is transformed from input digital display values, D, to display luminance L (see Fig. 3.7) with an approximately exponential relationship

$$L = L_{min}e^{KD}. \tag{3.1}$$

Using (Eq. 3.1), the display contrast is given by

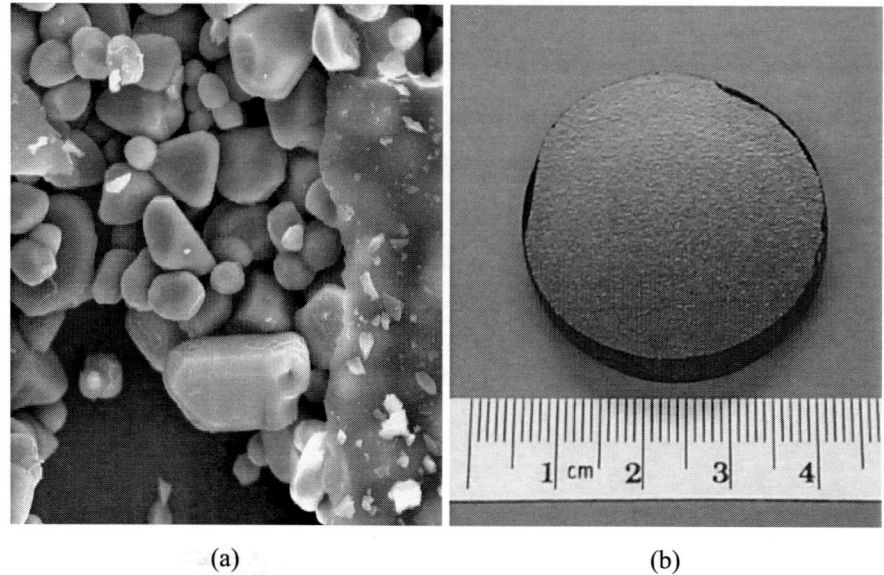

(a)   (b)

Figure 3.6 Components of the CRT emissive structure. Image (a) shows a scanning electron microscope image of a CRT face-plate sample. The phosphor layers were exposed using a scalpel scratch. The width of the image corresponds to 50 µm. Debris from the sample preparation process can be seen on top of the Al layer. Image (b) shows a CRT face-plate core showing the inner surface after removal of the phosphor and Al layers. The roughness in the interior surface contributes to diffusively scattered internal reflections. Reproduced from Ref. [61] with permission of the RSNA.

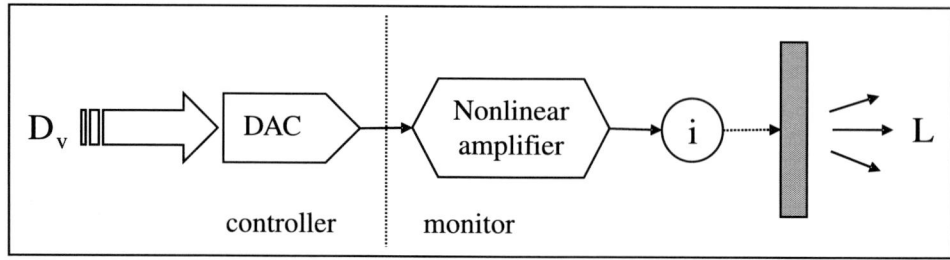

Figure 3.7 Transformation of the input signal from an image file (an array of D) into the luminance field in a CRT screen.

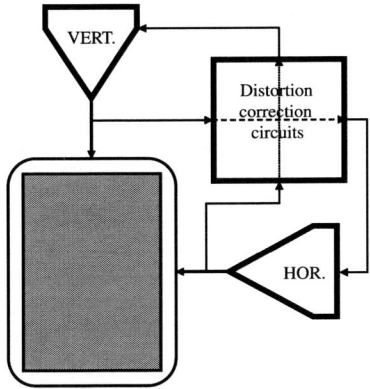

Figure 3.8 Deflection of the electron beam requires distortion-correction circuits to control beam focusing.

$$\frac{\Delta L}{L} = K\Delta D. \tag{3.2}$$

This internal transfer function that relates the gray-scale values to the output luminance is affected by the calibration procedure via a look-up table, which provides correction factors to adjust the response to a desired luminance response function.

Horizontal and vertical deflection amplifiers control the position of the electron beam for one or two image frames (see Fig. 3.8). The signal amplifier must have sufficient bandwidth to allow precise rendering of all the pixels in the image and to produce sharp graphics and text. When an image is displayed on the screen, the scanning electron beam modulates its intensity according to the gray-scale values representing the image. If large changes in image values (which will be translated into large changes in beam current and luminance output) are present, the electronics should be capable of modulating the beam with a time constant smaller than the time needed for the beam to excite the phosphor at that pixel location. Therefore, the bandwidth requirements for different pixel formats used in medical imaging workstations, shown in Table 3.1, depend on the pixel format. For instance, when displaying images at 80 MHz, a CRT with five Mpixels will require a deflection amplifier with 200 MHz for one frame per image, or 100 MHz for two frames per image.

Table 3.1 Bandwidth (in MHz) required at the deflection amplifiers.

80-MHz Display	Image	Graphics
2 Mpixels, 1 frame	80	320
2 Mpixels, 2 frames	40	160
5 Mpixels, 1 frame	200	400
5 Mpixels, 2 frames	100	200

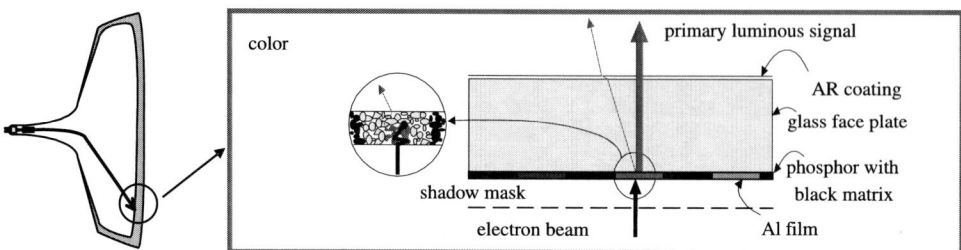

Figure 3.9 Emissive structure of a color CRT. For comparison with a monochrome CRT structure, see Fig. 3.5.

3.5 Color CRTs

Color CRTs differ significantly in their emissive structure (see Fig. 3.9) and typically have a lower display image quality when compared to monochrome CRTs. In any of the current main design alternatives (shadow mask or aperture grille), the emissive structure contains a black matrix that separates the three phosphor materials to form an arrangement of color dots or stripes (see Fig. 3.10). In addition to increasing the degradation in contrast by veiling glare (see Sec. 2.6), the light and electron scattering processes that take place within the emissive structure also reduce the color saturation (see Fig. 3.11). Color purity is obtained by increasing optical absorption in the emissive structure and by reducing electronic glare using low backscattering materials as mask coatings.[52, 161, 162]

Incorrect beam landing is a major concern in color CRTs due to the presence of the mask or grille. If mislanding occurs—that is, if the center of the electron beam does not fall in line with the center of the phosphor dot—then color purity is

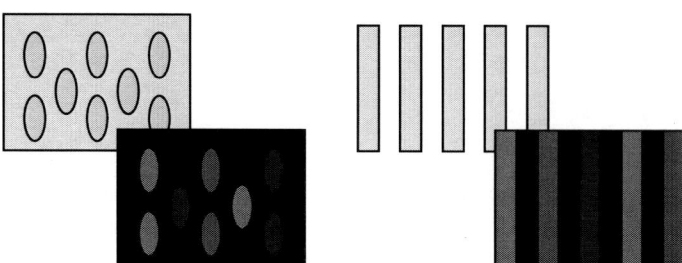

Figure 3.10 Designs for achieving color in a CRT. The shadow mask on the left is a perforated sheet placed in proximity to the phosphor screen to delimit the electron beam that hits the phosphor. Masks generally have higher electronic veiling glare due to the large fraction of backscattered electrons rejected from the primary beam. The aperture grille design on the right provides a higher aperture area for beam transmission while maintaining good definition between the color stripes.

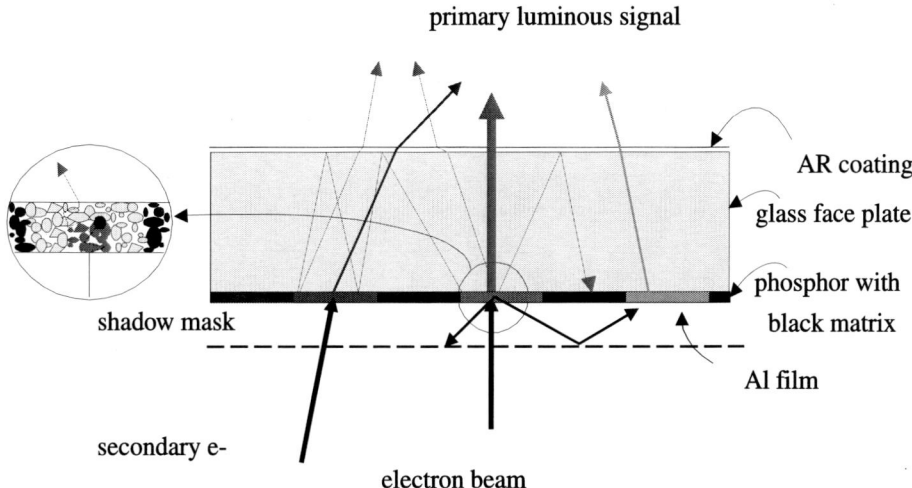

primary luminous signal

AR coating

glass face plate

phosphor with
black matrix

shadow mask

Al film

secondary e-

electron beam

Figure 3.11 Degradation of luminance and color contrast in a color CRT caused by optical and electron transport processes in the emissive structure.

degraded. In these designs, alignment of the electron beam with the openings of the mask or aperture grille is paramount, and color electron guns often compensate for the aberrations and space-charge effects that would degrade the convergence of the beam.

3.6 Spot Size

The electron spot size is typically defined as the width of the spot at 50% of the maximum luminance. At low luminance, spot sizes vary from 0.15–0.20 mm, while at high luminance, spot sizes increase to 0.15–0.30 mm. The width at 5% of the maximum is typically about twice the width at 50%.

The width of the spot is not constant across the screen, but increases at the edges relative to the center. To achieve well-defined spots, a high-frequency response is needed for sharp graphics (400 MHz at 3 db). In addition, a dynamic focus adjustment at the center and at the periphery using deflection information can greatly improve the resolution characteristics of the monitor. Tables 3.2 and 3.3 show spot sizes for different screen configurations.

Table 3.2   Beam spot size for a 300 × 400-mm field with a 50% overlap.

Number of Mpixels	Array Size	Spot Size (mm)
1	900 × 1100	0.35
2	1200 × 1600	0.25
5	2000 × 2700	0.15

Table 3.3   Beam spot size for a 270 × 330-mm field with a 50% overlap.

Number of Mpixels	Array Size	Spot Size (mm)
1	900 × 1100	0.3
2	1200 × 1600	0.21
5	2000 × 2700	0.13

3.7 Monochrome Phosphors

The choice of phosphor for a monochrome CRT is an important element to consider when comparing different monitors. Typically, two alternatives exist: a single-component phosphor (P45) or a blended phosphor (P104). P104 phosphors have higher luminous efficiency[*] but are made from a mixture of different-colored phosphors, which causes a granular appearance. On the other hand, P45 is a single-component phosphor with reduced granularity (see Fig. 6.17). The luminous efficiency of P45 is about 0.65 of P104's luminance efficiency. These figures come into play when considering the long-term use of the display because of aging effects due to coulomb loading, a term used to describe the amount of electron energy deposited into the phosphor grains. Phosphors degrade over time due to material changes in regions of high electron bombardment and high current density, resulting in a corresponding decrease in brightness. The user will need to correct for this decrease in brightness over the lifetime of the monitor. The relative magnitude of this effect for P45 and P104 is shown in Fig. 3.12. At 25 kV, and for an area of 1200 cm^2 with a luminance of 300 cd/m^2, a P104 phosphor is able to sustain a current density of 0.166 μA/cm^2 with a total of 1673 hours per coulomb deposited. Meanwhile, under the same conditions, a P45 screen will sustain 0.255 μA/cm^2 with a total of 1089 hours per coulomb.

---

[*]   Luminous efficiency is defined as the percentage of luminance compared to a standard phosphor (P4) under specified conditions of beam current, high voltage, and face-plate transmission. In an absolute scale, it is typically expressed in lm/watt.

3.8 Antireflection Surface Treatments

Medical monitors of good quality have a thin-film surface coating that provides three benefits: (a) conduction to eliminate static charge and reduce dust collection, (b) abrasion resistance, and (c) antireflection (AR) properties. It has also been shown that AR coatings reduce veiling glare in CRTs.[13] Coatings generally have many thin-film layers and are often laminated as added glass thickness to the display surface. Current multilayer designs are effective in reducing the specular component of the display reflectance (as shown in Fig. 3.13) without sacrificing brightness or adding unwanted color shifts.

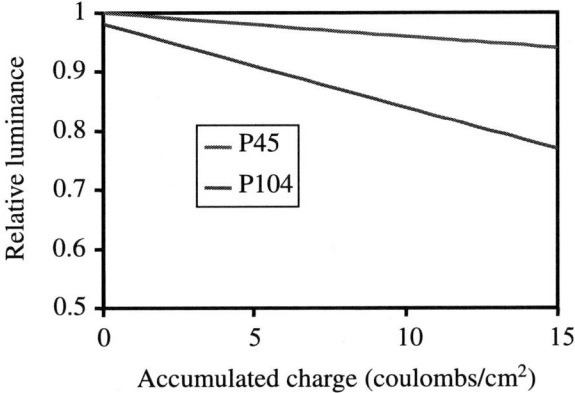

Figure 3.12 Reduction of the display luminance due to phosphor aging for P45 and P104 monochrome phosphors.

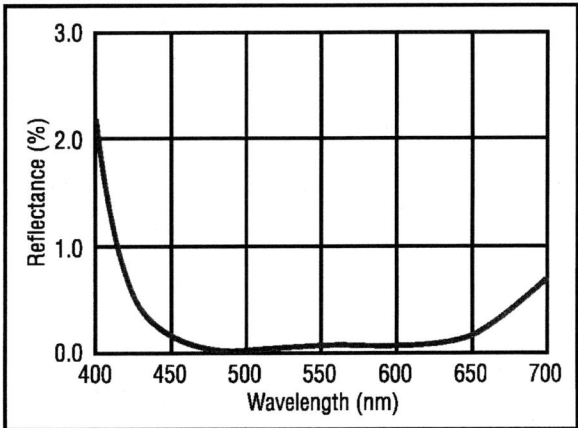

Figure 3.13 Antireflection properties of a multilayer thin-film coating used in medical imaging CRT monitors. Reprinted with permission from JDS Uniphase, Thin Film Products Group (formerly OCLI).

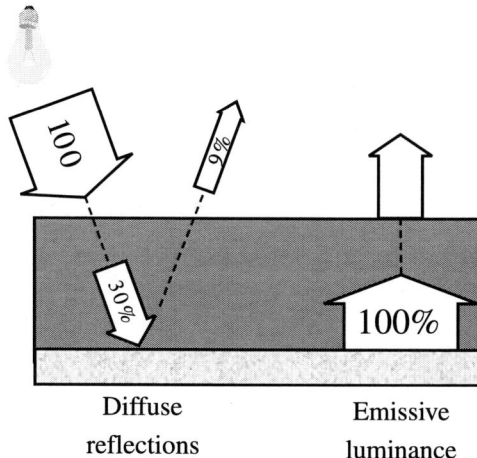

Diffuse

reflections

Emissive

luminance

Figure 3.14 Reduction of ambient light reflections using tinted glass. Absorptive glass reduces scattered light coming from ambient lights and from internal veiling glare. Reproduced from Ref. [6] with permission of the RSNA.

3.9 Face-plate Absorption

Light transmission through the face plate of medical monitors is typically 20–50% to reduce reflections from ambient light. If we assume a transmission of 30%, the diffuse reflections are reduced by at least 9%, resulting in improved black levels. Meanwhile, the display brightness only diminishes by 30% (see Fig. 3.14). The glass absorption also reduces veiling glare by dampening the optical scattering within the face plate.[13]

3.10 Gray-scale Controllers

The accuracy of a gray-scale presentation is affected by the quality of the display controller. The digital-to-analog converter (DAC) in the display controller determines its ability to modify the shape of the luminance response. Conventional controllers with an 8-bit DAC have limited control over the slope ($\Delta L/L$) of the display curve. Figure 3.15 shows the relative contrast at each of the first 20 gray levels for 8-, 9-, and 10-bit controllers. When an 8-bit DAC is utilized at the input and at the output of the conversion process, several gray-level steps occur without a corresponding change in the luminance output. When a 10-bit DAC is used, the number of unchanging gray levels is minimized. Controllers intended for medical applications are available with a 10-bit DAC from a variety of manufacturers.

The Digital Display Working Group (DDWG) was organized by a number of companies to define specifications for digital display connections. The DDWG (www.ddwg.org) is an industry group led by Intel that includes Compaq, Fujitsu,

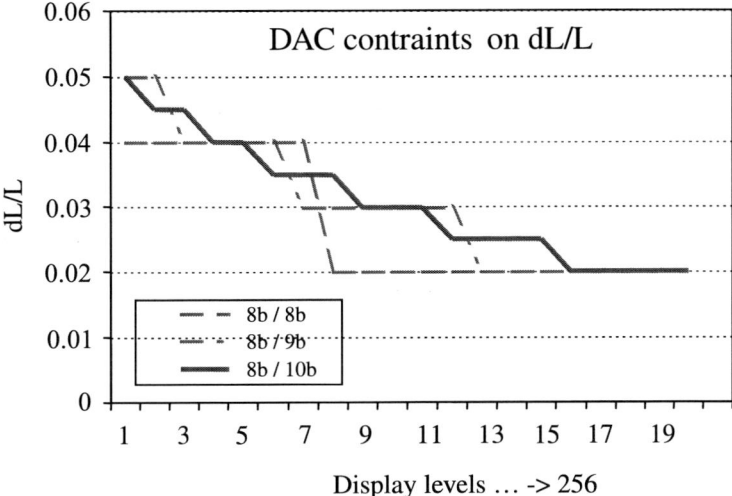

Figure 3.15 The precision of a gray-scale presentation is affected by the controller's bit depth. Digital-to-analog converters with higher bit depth provide a smoother transition between gray levels.

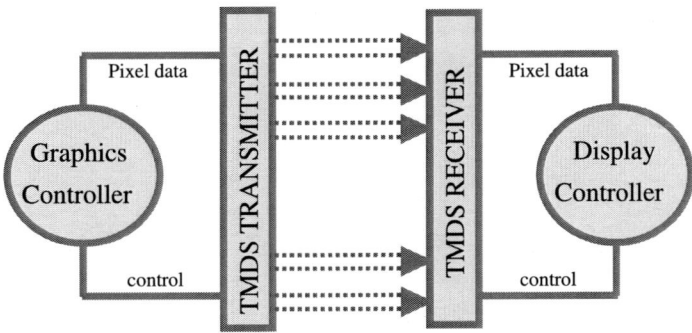

Figure 3.16 The digital video interface (DVI) transition-minimized differential signaling (TMDS) layers between the graphics controller and the display controller. TMDS links are used in existing AMLCD digital interfaces and in digital CRT monitors.

Hewlett Packard, IBM, NEC, and Silicon Image whose objective is to address the industry's requirements for digital connectivity in high-performance computing and digital displays. The DDWG specifications published in April 1999 endorsed Silicon Image's PanelLink technology for transition-minimized differential signaling (TMDS) and provided the technical basis for the proposed interface specification (see Fig. 3.16). It consists of a standardized connector with either a single-link mode (165 Mpixels/sec, 2 Mpixels at 82 Hz) or a dual-link mode (330 Mpixels/sec, 4 Mpixels at 82 Hz). The standard applies to CRTs and flat-panel displays (FPDs), and bridges the gap between analog and digital interfaces.

Chapter 4
Active-Matrix
Liquid Crystal Displays

I am at a loss to give a distinct idea of the nature of this liquid, and cannot do so without many words. Although it flowed with rapidity in all declivities where common water would do so, yet never, except when falling in a cascade, had it the customary appearance of limpidity. It was, nevertheless, in point of fact, as perfectly limpid as any limestone water in existence, the difference being only in appearance. At first sight, and especially in cases where little declivity was found, it bore resemblance, as regards consistency, to a thick infusion of gum arabic in common water. But this was only the least remarkable of its extraordinary qualities.

—Edgar Allan Poe, in an excerpt from *The Narrative of Arthur Gordon Pym of Nantucket* (1850)

This chapter introduces the basic technological aspects of liquid crystal displays (LCDs) and provides an overall perspective on LCD characteristics, with an emphasis on the design elements that affect image quality. After a brief review of liquid crystal technology, we describe many aspects related to the design of AMLCD monitors used in medical imaging systems.

Liquid crystal (LC) is an intermediate state of matter that possesses properties typical of solids (i.e., a crystalline structure with a highly ordered molecular arrangement), as well as properties associated with liquids (i.e., viscosity).[45] LC materials are typically long organic molecules with a delocalized charge due to multiple unsaturated bonds and aromatic rings. Because of this charge delocalization, molecules are electrically polarized, forming strong dipoles. Most importantly, LC molecules tend to orient themselves loosely along a main axis (called a *director*) to form a unique spatial configuration determined by the elasticity, viscosity, and deformation constants.

4.1 The Liquid Crystal Cell

Many LC cell types can be generated with different cell configurations. The most common configurations are shown in Fig. 4.1(a). The degree of alignment of LC molecules is often characterized by the order parameter S, given by the following expression

$$S = \frac{1}{2} < 3\cos^2\theta - 1 >, \tag{4.1}$$

where θ is the angle between each individual LC molecule and the director orientation, and $< >$ denotes the average over all molecules. The spatial arrangement of the LC molecules leads to anisotropy, a characteristic defined as the dependence of the material properties on the direction of measurement.

In order to make use of LC properties to modulate light transmission, the orientation of LC molecules needs to be controlled. When LC molecules encounter a textured surface, they align parallel to the grooves [see Fig. 4.1(a)]. By applying cross rubbing directions in the top and bottom plates, LC molecules can be oriented in a way that creates a twist along the cell [Fig. 4.1(b)]. The fundamental discovery that led to display applications of LCs[51, 92] is the finding that the director can be altered by an external electric field. Figure 4.2 shows an example of the change in LC arrangement that occurs when an electric field is applied between the top and bottom electrodes.

When the director is twisted, light polarization also twists due to the birefringence in the LC layer. In the example of Fig. 4.2, the twist is exactly 90 deg. The wavelength dependence of this effect leads to slightly colored panels when white backlight is used. With the help of polarizer films that allow transmission of light when the polarization vector and the axis of the film are aligned, LC cells can be designed to transmit or block light when a pixel voltage is applied. When the twist in the LC director and the configuration of top and bottom polarizer films are such

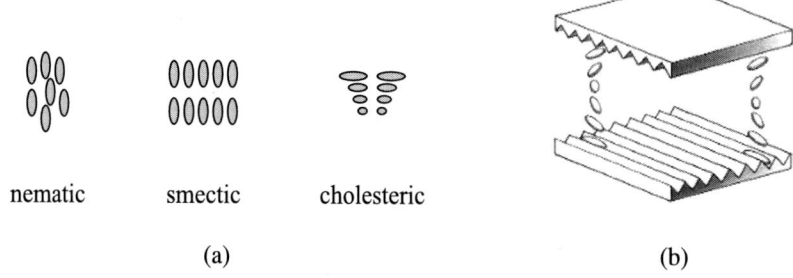

nematic   smectic   cholesteric

(a)   (b)

Figure 4.1 Alignment of LC molecules along the main molecular axis, called the director. (a) Different configurations of LC cells with respect to the director orientation and their generic names. (b) Alignment of LC molecules along rubbing directions to generate a twist in the display cell.

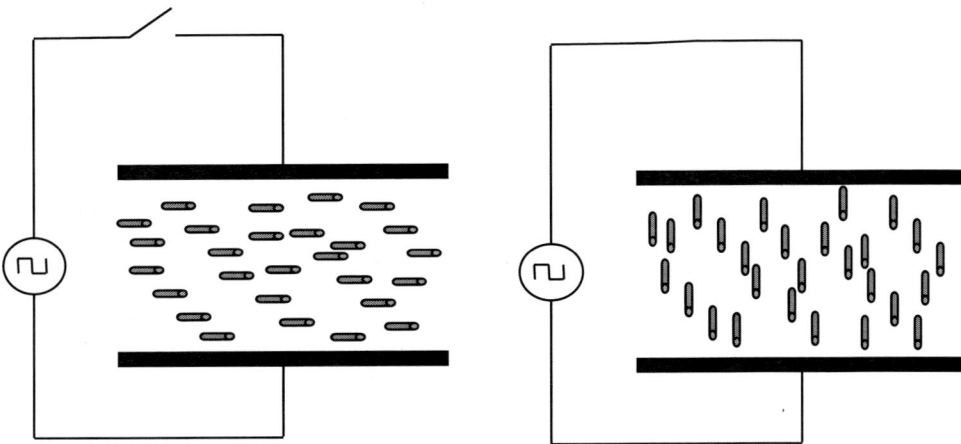

Figure 4.2 Change in LC orientation due to an external electric field applied between the top and bottom electrodes.

that light is fully transmitted with no applied voltage, the LC cell is called *normally white*. When light is blocked in these conditions, we have a *normally black* cell. A schematic plot of light transmission as a function of applied cell voltage is shown in Fig. 4.3. As shown in Fig. 4.4, a number of elements are required to achieve the electro-optical effect responsible for gray-scale control.

In addition to the top and bottom substrates, alignment layers, polarizer films, and electrodes, spacers are needed to maintain a given thickness in the LC cell. The accuracy with which the cell thickness (typically in the order of a few microns) is controlled has direct implications on the luminance variations across the LCD screen. Typically, spherical glass beads (with or without absorbers) are used as spacers by spraying them on the bottom plate before introduction of the LC material.

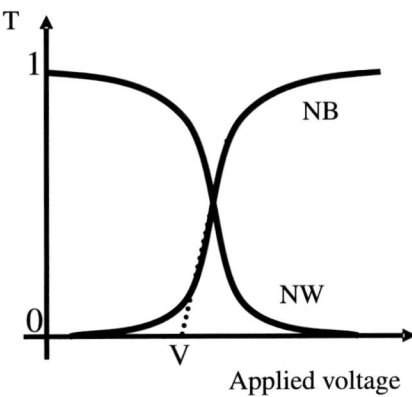

Figure 4.3 The LC electro-optical effect that defines light transmission (T) as a function of applied cell voltage for a *normally white* (NW) and *normally black* (NB) device. V_{th} is the threshold voltage at which the LC molecules are realigned.

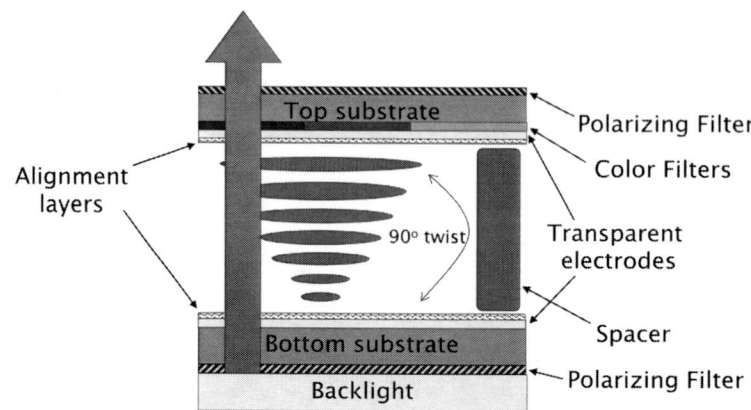

Figure 4.4 Elements of a typical LCD.

4.2 Efficiency of Light Transmission

Because of the multitude of elements that light needs to go through before generating an image in the front screen, LCDs are intrinsically inefficient devices. Typically, only 3–5% of the total light generated by the backlight is seen on the front face of a color LCD. This fraction is higher for monochrome devices (on the order of 8–15%) due to their lack of color filters, which absorb much of the light in color devices. A schematic representation of the reduction in luminance as light traverses the LCD is presented in Fig. 4.5. The percentages refer to transmitted luminance and are dependent on the optical performance of the layers.

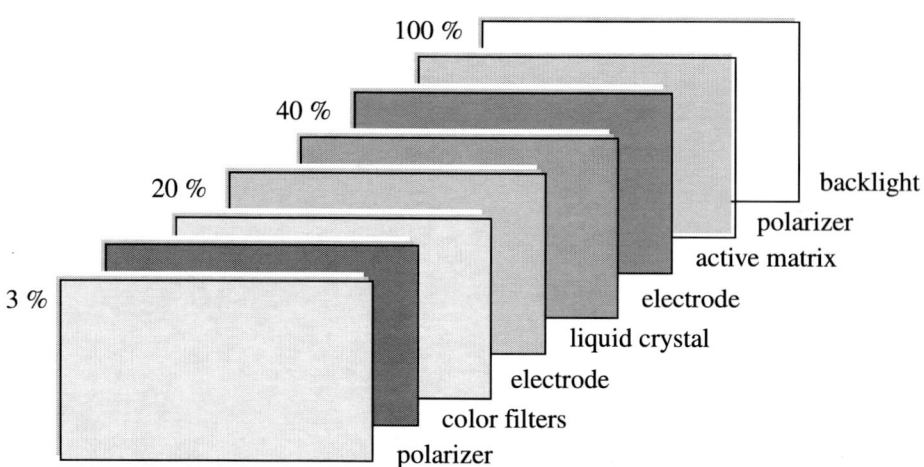

Figure 4.5 Power efficiency and brightness reduction as light passes through the multiple layers of an AMLCD. In color systems, the RGB color filters cause a significant reduction in luminance.

Given the transmission of typical LC stacks, a highly efficient backlight is needed. A backlight consists of one or many multiple-phosphor lamps, a reflector, and a diffuser. The critical design parameters are compactness, efficiency, and life expectancy. In LCD applications, both behind-the-panel (brighter) or on-edge (better uniformity and small thickness) designs have been developed. Typical lifetimes are 10,000 h for a hot cathode fluorescent tube (HCFT) and 20,000 h for a cold cathode fluorescent tube (CCFT).

Another means to increase efficiency of the LC transmission is by employing high-quality polarizer films. These are typically iodine-doped polymer films stretched in one direction. The oriented polymer chains substituted with iodine generate uneven electron densities and selective light absorption or even extinction for a given light polarization direction (up to 99% in degree of polarization at the output of the films). A major cause of luminance loss in color LCDs is the RGB color filters used to obtain full color. Typically, each pixel is divided into three subpixels with a red, green, or blue filter on top. The color filters can be formed by patterning and dyeing resin deposits, by pigment impregnation, or by printing.

4.3 Addressing Methods

The control of pixel luminance is achieved using a variety of techniques by controlling the voltage at each individual LC cell that represents an LCD pixel. The most simple of these techniques is called static drive. In a static addressing technique, one side has only one connector per pixel, and the other side has a common electrode (see top of Fig. 4.6). In contrast, an active drive requires a switch at each pixel (see bottom of Fig. 4.6).

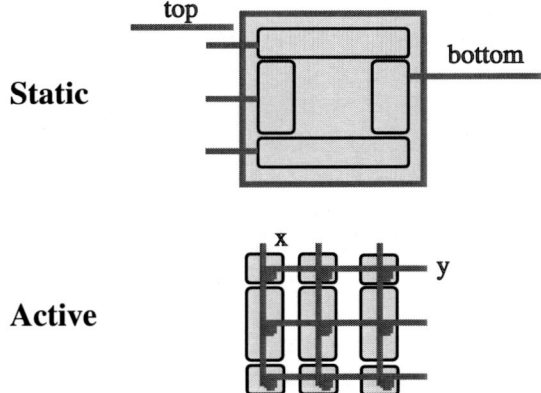

Figure 4.6 Addressing methods for AMLCDs: a static technique (top) uses only one common electrode, while an active technique (bottom) requires a switching device (typically a thin-film transistor or TFT) at each pixel.

The disadvantages of using passive addressing are most notable in high-resolution displays. As the number of rows and columns increases (higher pixel density), the electrode size must be reduced and the voltage necessary to passively drive the display increases. The higher driving voltage creates, in turn, more severe parasitic effects. In this scenario, the voltage setting of a central pixel significantly affects adjacent LC cells, reducing the display contrast by partially activating surrounding pixels. In addition, the time frame for passive matrix (PM) is slow (150–300 ms).

Most commonly used in high-resolution LCDs, addressing of the individual pixels is performed using an active matrix (AM). An AM can be considered as an array of nearly ideal switches (fast transition from the "black" state to full transmission of an LC cell). This provides for faster and more accurate control of the pixel gray level. The performance required in the AM depends on the display performance requirements and on the spatial and gray-scale resolution. A more detailed description of the AM is given in the next section.

4.4 Elements of an AMLCD

The worldwide market for displays has evolved rapidly in recent years. Panel sizes and resolution levels have grown significantly while prices have diminished considerably. Between 1997 and 2002, the market sales for LCDs (including passively and actively addressed) increased from $13 million to $30 million. During the same period, AMLCDs experienced an increase from $8 million to $23 million. Although sales of LCDs for portable computers dominated the market in 1997, they were comparable to the sales for desktop applications during 2001 and are likely to recede in years to come. At the same time, the size of most commercialized LCDs increased from about 12 inches in 1998 to about 15 inches in 2002.[119]

Due to this trend in overall display markets, we are now experiencing the availability of high-resolution AMLCD monitors manufactured for demanding applications such as satellite and medical imaging. In the remainder of this chapter, we describe current designs of monochrome AMLCDs that are being sought for the medical imaging markets with an emphasis on the design features that are most relevant for their successful introduction into the radiology practice.

As explained in the previous section, an AMLCD consists of a stack of layers, each serving a particular purpose. Figure 4.7 shows a typical AMLCD assembly in which light travels from the rear polarizer filter through the color filters, the back and front plates, and the LC cells until light is finally emitted at the front face plate. All the elements in this figure are present in any LC design, regardless of the particular arrangement of the LC molecules as defined by the display's LC mode.[51, 92]

One of the principal components of the AMLCD monitor is the switch in the AM array responsible for pixel addressing. In AMLCDs, this element is usually a thin-film transistor (TFT). The most commonly used TFT technology in AMLCDs is amorphous silicon (a-Si:H). Table 4.1 presents some of the advantages and disadvantages of the a-Si:H technology[41] compared to the polycrystalline Si (p-Si)

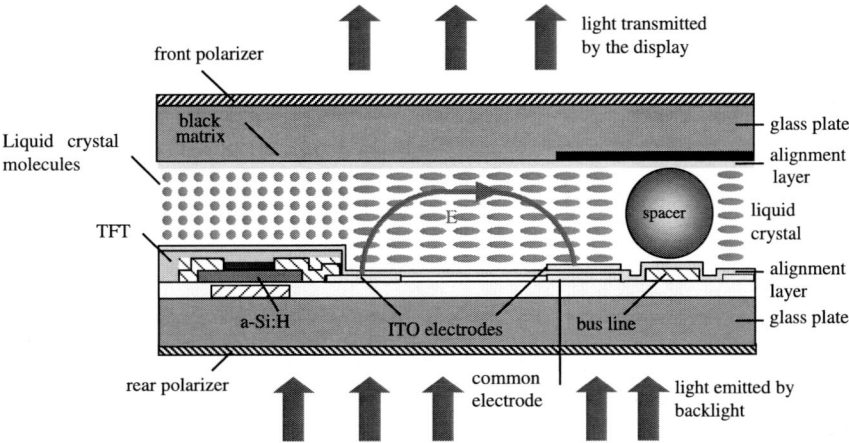

Figure 4.7 Cross section of a color AMLCD showing typical components. Reproduced from Ref. [6] with permission of the RSNA.

approach. Although a much greater mobility can be achieved with the p-Si, the a-Si:H has the most important advantage of being a mature technology that has proven itself in manufacturing plants where large-area substrates are processed at low temperatures. A fundamental characteristic of the TFT design is the ON/OFF current ratio that the transistor is capable of. Figure 4.8 shows a typical curve of drain-source current as a function of the voltage applied between the gate and the source. This particular design has a low leakage current that satisfies the requirements for high-definition display systems.[125]

The TFTs are usually located on one of the corners of the display pixel, as shown in Fig. 4.9. Since the TFT circuitry is shielded from the high illumination coming from the backlight by an opaque coating, light is not transmitted over the area where the TFT is deposited. The fraction of the total pixel area that allows transmission of light is called the *aperture ratio*. In consumer product displays,

Table 4.1 TFT technologies used for AMLCDs.

Parameter	a-Si:H	p-Si
Mobility (cm^2/V.s)	0.6–1.5	50–100
Size (µm)	Micron	Submicron
Drivers	Separate	Integrated
Cost	Cheap	Expensive
Processing temperature	Low	High
Other	Reliable over large areas	High resolution Faster response

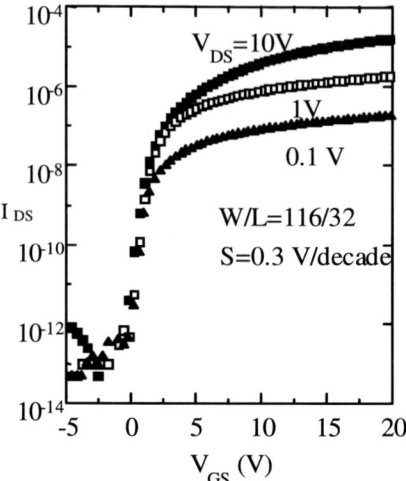

Figure 4.8   Typical a-Si:H TFT response curve with high ON/OFF ratio.

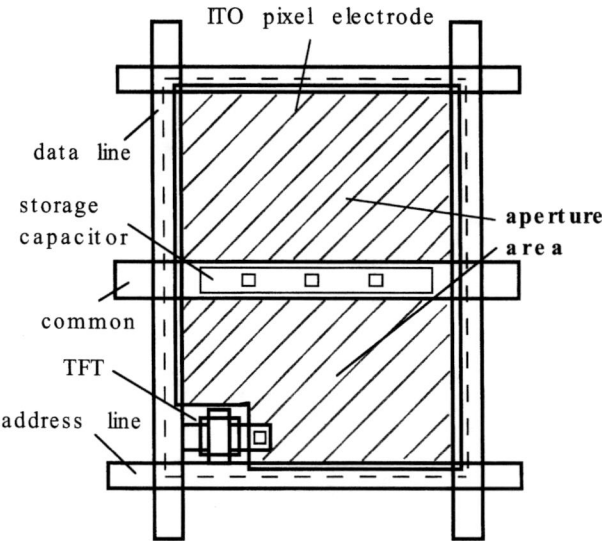

Figure 4.9   Pixel layout defining the aperture ratio and the TFT with associated circuitry. Reprinted from Ref. [61] with permission of the RSNA.

the aperture ratio can be as small as 50%, while in high-performance displays it can be as high as 80%. The aperture ratio affects the display power requirements and the control of the luminance levels. For instance, in a 10.4-in. SVGA display, the power can be reduced by a factor of 0.57 due to an enhanced aperture ratio. A higher aperture ratio also increases the achievable display contrast performance by reducing the nonactive regions or gaps of the display pixel.

One method to improve aperture ratio is to reduce the indium tin oxide (ITO) pixel electrode to bus line separation. Figure 4.9 shows a TFT design with overlap between the ITO and the bus lines (data lines). As the gate signal reaches the other end of the gate line, it suffers a time constant of about $\tau = RC$. This delay limits display size and resolution. For large-area, high-resolution displays, Cu or Al metallization should be used.[94, 104]

4.5 Crosstalk in AMLCDs

Due to the thin face plate that AMLCDs and FPDs commonly have, these display devices do not suffer from veiling glare.[9] However, the manner in which the AM addresses the individual pixels through row and column circuits introduces another mechanism for contrast reduction commonly referred to as *crosstalk*. The effect of crosstalk is seen as a change in the pixel luminance of the displayed image in a region where there is a significant change in the gray level across the vertical or horizontal directions, as shown in Fig. 4.10(a).

In AMLCDs, the voltage applied across the LC cell through the pixel electrodes defines the pixel luminance. Crosstalk is associated with the unwanted modification of the pixel voltage effectively applied to the LC cell because of incomplete pixel charging, leakage currents in the TFT, and parasitic capacitive coupling. Accordingly, display crosstalk is more important in large-size panels with high spatial and gray-scale resolution.[108, 109] Although having different origins, crosstalk artifacts have also been studied for PM organic polymer light-emitting displays (OLEDs).[33] In large array sizes, parasitic capacitances in the long

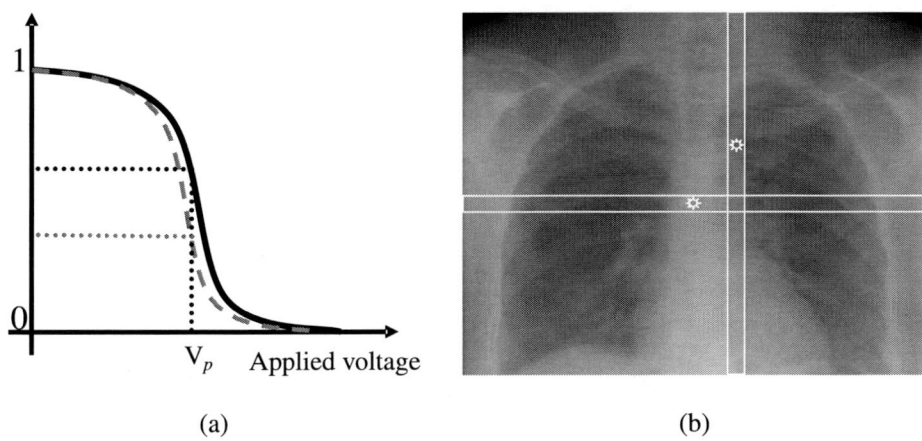

(a)   (b)

Figure 4.10 Effect of crosstalk on a displayed image. In (a), the change in pixel voltage, V_p, determines a change in light transmission from T_p to T'_p. The solid curve represents the desired applied voltage. The dashed curve is the actual pixel voltage. Crosstalk reduces the display contrast in areas where large luminance changes occur along the column or row [see marked locations in (b)].

lines across the display screen give rise to unwanted modifications of the pixel voltage, affecting the accuracy of the gray level, as shown in Fig. 4.10(b).

In the AMLCD industry, crosstalk is known to have two components: optical and electronic. The optical crosstalk is generally a short-range effect with a characteristic distance of fewer than 10 display pixels, and is negligible at longer interaction distances. On the other hand, electronic crosstalk has complex spatial characteristics that depend strongly on orientation (vertical versus horizontal according to the panel wiring scheme). An electronic crosstalk artifact is not radially symmetric due to the matrix arrangement of the display circuitry. Moreover, the effect is not shift-invariant since leakage currents, photo-generated currents, and parasitic capacitances are not uniform across the display matrix.[15, 115] Proposed methods for the reduction of crosstalk employ modified driving techniques to maintain, to a certain extent, the desired pixel voltage at each individual pixel in the AM array.

4.6 Luminance Variations with Viewing Angle

Cathode-ray tubes and most emissive displays emit light in a way that the angular luminous intensity closely follows a cosine distribution. Consequently, the display luminance remains constant across all viewing directions. That is not the case for LCDs. In LCDs, the luminance and the contrast are a strong function of the viewing direction (see Fig. 4.11). In some AMLCDs, at high off-axis angles, the asymmetric variations can be severe enough to cause an inversion of the gray scale, a condition that is unacceptable in most diagnostic workstations.

Figures 4.12 and 4.13 present results for the luminance and contrast variations, respectively, for a typical medical imaging CRT and for an AMLCD. Both display systems have been calibrated using the DICOM gray-scale presentation

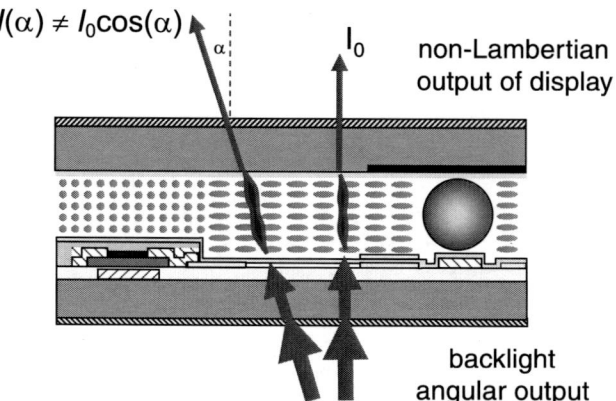

Figure 4.11 Cross section of an AMLCD showing two light paths corresponding to two different viewing directions. The different path lengths and spatial alignments with respect to the LC director configuration determines a different transmission through the LC cell.

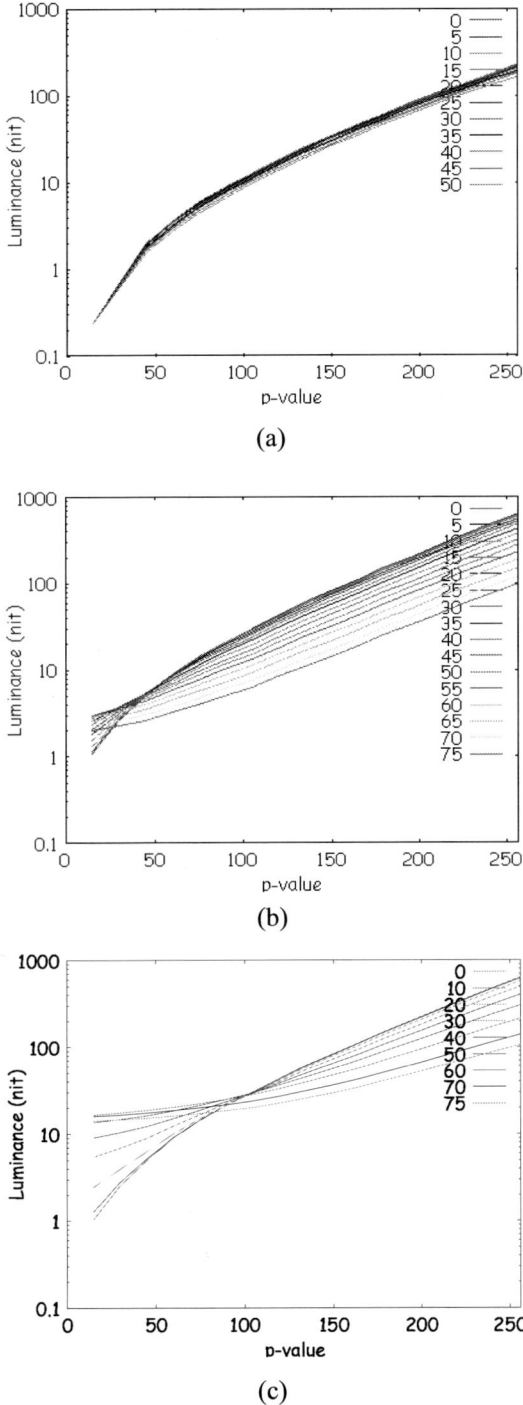

Figure 4.12 Display luminance curves as a function of the viewing direction for a medical imaging CRT (a), and for an AMLCD [(b) is in the horizontal direction, and (c) is in the diagonal direction].

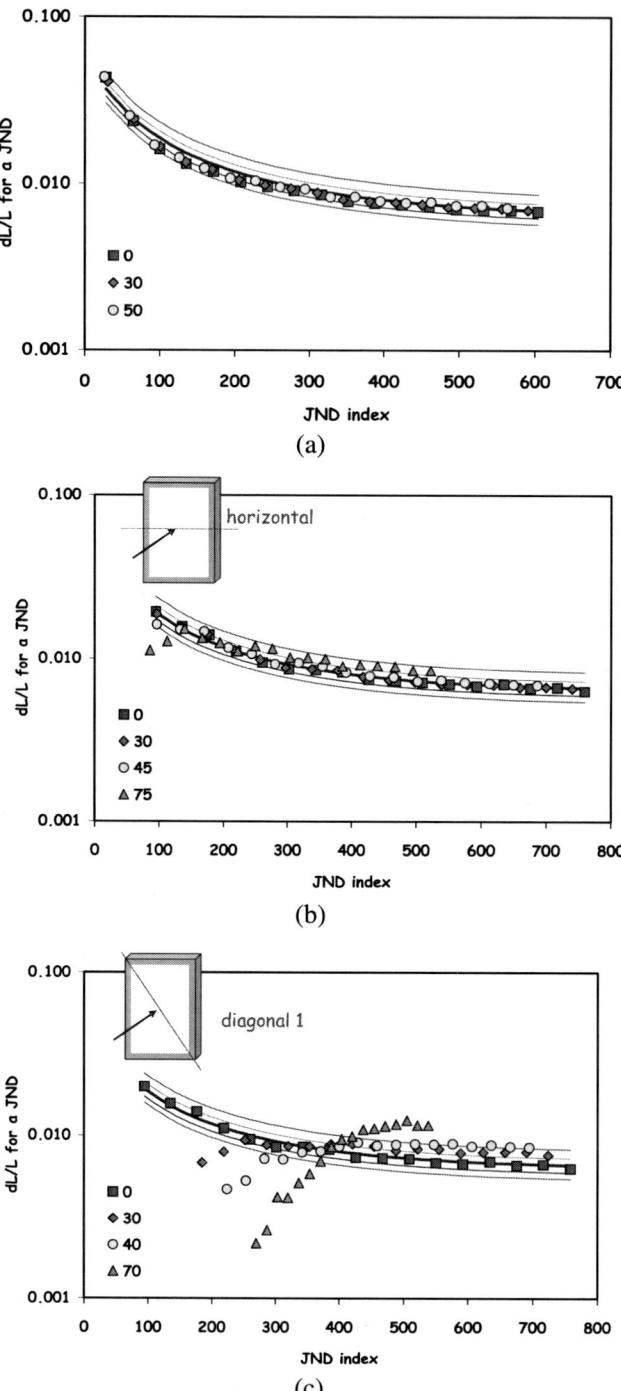

Figure 4.13 Display contrast expressed as dL/L as a function of the viewing direction for a medical imaging CRT (a), and for an AMLCD [(b) is in the horizontal direction, and (c) is in the diagonal direction].

function.[2] The luminance changes for the CRT monitor with viewing angle are small, and the corresponding changes in the contrast (associated with the slope of the luminance curve) are within 10% of the desired response. In the case of the AMLCD, the more dramatic changes in the luminance cause a significant reduction of the contrast in the low luminance regions, accompanied by a decrease in the available JNDs.

The implications of this problem in medical imaging monitors is twofold. First, a single user of the device will experience its effects when looking at different areas of the display screen, depending on the dimension of the screen surface (which can reach more than 30 cm in one of the sides). In this scenario, the more severe changes in the luminance presentation curve associated with the viewing angle are likely to happen between the center and the corners of the screen. The second aspect of this problem arises when more than one individual is looking at the same image displayed in the same screen. In this case, the variations are larger because of varying viewing angles and the departure from on-axis calibration.

4.7 Solutions to Viewing Angle Problem

Several solutions have been developed to compensate for the angular variations of display luminance. The approaches come from recognizing that the anisotropy of the light modulation is the dominating factor in defining the viewing angle characteristics of a device. When the light beams arrive at different angles with respect to the display surface normal, they experience different effective optical paths through the LC. This condition is more severe for an intermediate gray level, where the LC molecules are oriented in an oblique direction with respect to the display surface. The solutions that we describe in this text belong to three different classes: compensation films, multiple domains, and specially aligned LC arrangements.

Although these technologies significantly improve the viewing angle characteristics, some trade-offs exist in other display-quality parameters such as transmittance and brightness, and temporal response. None of these technologies by itself can satisfy the requirements in all areas of display image quality. In current AMLCD designs, many, if not all, of the three classes are combined and employed in a single device. The benefits of using one of these technologies are compounded with the addition of another. However, as we examine next, these technologies have drawbacks.

4.7.1 Compensation foils

Special birefringent films have been designed to compensate for the anisotropy introduced by the LC alignment with respect to the different directions of light transmitted by the LC cell.[82, 123] The films, called *foils*, ideally match the profile of the director in a given state (for a given pixel luminance) by counteracting the

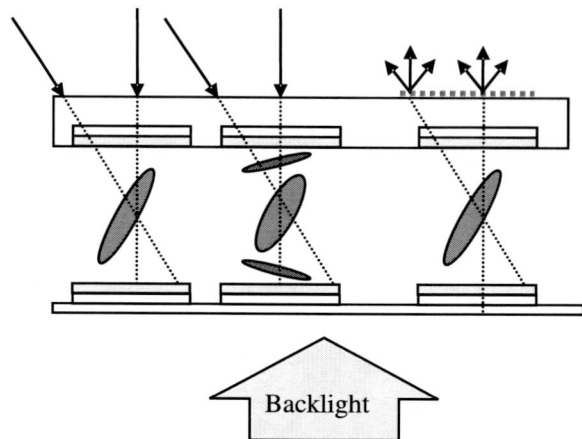

Figure 4.14 Compensation films can be used to improve the viewing angle of an AML-CD. On the center drawing, two birefringent films have been added (top and bottom) to the LC cell shown in the left. The electro-optical effect experienced by light travelling at different directions becomes more uniform at all angles. The far right drawing shows another approach that uses a diffuse film on top of the stack to redirect light paths. This solution provides good viewing angle characteristics, although the displayed image suffers from artifacts due to the microstructure of the diffuser.

birefringence of the LC layer. Since the films are static by not being dynamically adjustable with the pixel gray level, the compensation is optimal only for a single luminance level. One or two films in symmetrical configuration can be used to improve the compensation, as shown in Fig. 4.14.

4.7.2 Multiple domain cells

The viewing angle of an AMLCD can be significantly improved by dividing the pixel area into multiple subpixel domains having different orientational states of the LC molecules. Thus, the difference in viewing direction can be reduced since directionality of the molecule is not homogeneous when the electric field is applied.

The differential alignment of the LC is achieved by a sequence of conventional rubbing techniques on the alignment layer and photolithographic processes. Alternatively, the alignment can be achieved using selective patterning with polarized UV light treatment. Since each domain has an asymmetric response as a function of the viewing direction, the net effect is an average emission that tends to reduce the luminance variations with angle.

Two- and four-domain devices have been demonstrated, while eight-domain devices have been simulated.[42, 126] The main challenge associated with this technology is the domain stability associated with a highly changing director orientation across the small subpixel dimensions. In addition, the fabrication cost increases significantly with the number of domains due to the increase in processing steps.

4.7.3 Symmetry micro-cells

Yamada et al. have reported the axis symmetry micro-cell in which nematic liquid crystal is surrounded by polymer walls.[167] The symmetric micro-cells are fabricated by phase separation of LC and polymer. The polymer wall is fabricated by UV exposure. The chiral compound is added to nematic LC to realize a twisted orientation. The method not only has the advantage of a wide viewing angle due to the axis symmetry orientation but also no disclination due to mono-domain orientation. This leads to a wide viewing angle with high contrast.

4.7.4 In-plane switching

If the LC director remains in the display plane for all gray-scale states, the asymmetry for the different angles is minimized. This is implemented in the in-plane switching structure, where the pixel electrodes are located on the same bottom glass plate [see Fig. 4.15(a)]. The switching of the LC cell between on and off states comes from the application of an electric field parallel to the glass plates.[116, 164] In this method, the switch of the LC molecules is achieved using a lateral electric field. Because the LC molecules do not stand up diagonally, the variations of contrast with viewing angle are small. Although this improves the angular constancy of the luminance, it also reduces the transmission through the LC stack due to the presence of interdigitated electrodes.

In in-plane switching designs, the degradation of the display contrast is the most severe along the diagonal directions. This problem can be reduced by using wide viewing-angle polarizers or single- or dual-compensation plates.[43] Overall,

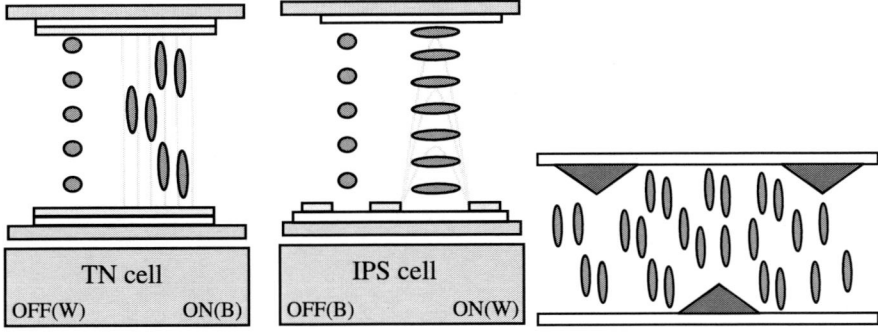

(a) In the IPS design, both pixel electrodes are located in the same plate, as opposed to the top and bottom plates in the twisted nematic (TN). The LC director remains in the display plane, improving the viewing angle.

(b) A schematic drawing of a vertically aligned LC cell with protrusions in both plates.

Figure 4.15 Advanced designs of LCD cells to reduce the change of luminance and contrast with viewing angle.

in-plane switching provides a wide viewing-angle solution with minimal grey-scale inversions and no major color shifts. The drawbacks of in-plane switching include low light efficiency due to the small aperture ratio, high driving voltages, and less reliability due to the more complex cell structure.

4.7.5 Vertical alignment

Contrary to the conventional TN method, high-contrast ratios can be obtained with vertical alignment because the molecular axis of an LC molecule is almost perpendicular to the substrate, and the black level is comparable to the characteristics of a cross-polarizer when no electric field is applied. In a normally black mode, a perfectly vertically aligned LC provides a near-perfect blockage of light when perpendicularly crossed polarizers are used. This arrangement can be achieved by oblique electrical fields with displaced electrodes, or, more commonly, with pyramid-shaped protrusions on both substrate plates [see Fig. 4.15(b)].[131] Excellent viewing angle characteristics have been reported in designs that combine vertical alignment with multiple domains. The capability to obtain high contrast and high response rates simultaneously is another feature of this method. Multiple vertical-aligned LCs have been proposed including multidomain VA (MVA), enhanced VA (EVA), and patterned VA (PVA). However, vertical alignment cannot completely solve the problem of gray-scale inversion, especially at high luminances.

Chapter 5
Active-Matrix Organic Light-Emitting Displays

The dream is thus to put electronic circuit properties into single molecules. Arrays of such molecules – possibly connected by conductive-polymer wires – on molecular scaffoldings would form molecular wafers. One may speculate that reduced dimensions from 200 nm to, say, 2 Å, and the concomitant shrinkage in circuit size could increase the speed and dynamic memory of computers by a factor of 108. Such progress would correspond to forty years of computer technology development. Conductive polymers may become crucial for the building of such a molecular electronics world.

—B. Nordé and E. Krutmeijer in the announcement of the 2000 Nobel Prize in Chemistry to A. J. Heeger, A. G. MacDiarmid, and H. Shirakawa, for the discovery and development of electrically conductive polymers

5.1 Introduction to OLEDs

Organic light-emitting devices (OLEDs) are one of the most rapidly developing technologies in recent FPD history. Since the first appearance of OLEDs in the market as a monochromatic car stereo display in 1997, tremendous research from academia and industry has been performed to implement OLED-based display for low-cost, small to medium, FPD applications.[120] According to the OLED display industry's 2003 report of Stanford Resources and Strategies Unlimited, the worldwide OLED display market is expected to increase up to $2 billion (U.S.) by 2006.

OLEDs have several advantages over other FPD technologies: their Lambertian self-emission property[105] produces a wide viewing angle; their fast response time (below microseconds) is a benefit for moving images; their high luminous efficiency and low operation voltage guarantee low power consumption by the display; their lightweight, very thin structure and robustness against external impacts are desirable characteristics for portable display applications; their simple, low-temperature fabrication process is cost effective; and their thin-film conformability on plastic substrates renders them a promising candidate for flexible display applications.[1, 88] Furthermore, when OLEDs are driven by an AM driving scheme based on TFTs, they can be used in high-resolution, large-size FPD applications such as laptop computers and TV screens. Recently, many companies—Toshiba and Matsushita,[158] Kodak and Sanyo,[101] Sony,[156] Samsung SDI,[145] and Chi Mei Optoelectronics and IBM Japan[159] have reported 15- to 24-in. active-matrix organic light-emitting display (AMOLED) prototypes with wide eXtended graphics array (WXGA) at 1200×768 resolution or eXtended graphics array (XGA) at 1024×768 resolution. The specifications of these prototypes are summarized in Table 5.1.

Table 5.1 Specifications of AMOLED prototypes.

Specification	Manufacturer				
	Toshiba and Matsushita	Kodak and Sanyo	Sony	Samsung SDI	Chi Mei Opto-electronics and IBM Japan
Screen Size (in.)	17	15	24.2	15.5	20
Resolution	WXGA/ 1280×768	WXGA/ 1280×720	XGA/ 1024×768	WXGA/ 1280×768	WXGA/ 1280×768
TFT Technology	poly-silicon	poly-silicon	poly-silicon	poly-silicon	amorphous silicon
Peak Brightness	300 cd/m^2	N/A	> 200 cd/m^2	N/A	500 cd/m^2
Emissive Material	polymer	small molecule	small molecule	small molecule	small molecule

5.1.1 History of OLEDs

Electroluminescence (EL) is the process of causing light emission from the radiative recombination of electrically created electrons and holes in organic materials. The discovery of EL of organic crystals can be dated back to the 1960s.[136] However, these early EL devices utilizing organic materials required several hundred volts and the light emission was inefficient.

During the late 1970s and early 1980s, the EL of organic thin films was advanced by reducing the operating voltage down to several tens of volts. This was achieved by subliming organic thin-films in a vacuum and using metal oxide electrodes.[139, 163] The efficiency of EL in organic materials was further improved by new device configurations and new emissive materials. A charge-transport layer was inserted between the electrodes and the emissive material. Tang and Van Slyke observed efficient green light emission from 8-hydroxyquinoline aluminum (Alq_3) by inserting a hole-transporting layer (HTL) of aromatic diamine between the active material and the transparent ITO electrode.[155] In the 1990s, polymeric materials gained wide attention as strong candidates for light-emitting materials. Electroluminescence was observed in a layer of poly (phenylene vinylene) (PPV) sandwiched between two metallic electrodes when the device was sufficiently biased.[36] The EL in polymeric materials is from the radiative recombination of the singlet exciton across the π-π^* energy gap. Greenham et al. made a major breakthrough by inserting another polymer layer[69] having a band mismatch with the active polymer layer, causing the injected carriers to be trapped at the interface and resulting in an efficient charge recombination with a 20-fold enhancement of device quantum efficiency.

Overall, significant progress in OLEDs has been achieved in the last decade. Material advancement has enabled fabrication of white light,[98] blue light,[106] variable color,[26] and polarized EL devices.[53] The efficiency of OLEDs has also gained from material engineering. Typical examples include the use of phosphorescent organic material to enhance the internal quantum efficiency and the use of electrostatically self-assembled multilayers to reduce the hole injection barrier height for efficient carrier injection.[17, 81]

5.1.2 OLEDs for displays

After decades of research, OLEDs have exceeded their inorganic counterparts in light-emission performance. The light emission from OLEDs covers the full visible spectrum. They are inexpensive to fabricate and can be patterned on both planar and flexible substrates. Current research on LEDs made from organic semiconductors has shown high brightness and high power-conversion efficiency. Furthermore, displays made using OLEDs overcome many disadvantages associated with traditional LCDs. As discussed in Chapter 4, the disadvantages of LCDs include a narrow viewing angle and a slow response time of the LC molecules. Because OLEDs are emissive devices, components such as the backlight, polarizers, and top glass necessary in LCDs are not needed in OLED displays. OLED displays have a wide viewing angle, high brightness and contrast ratio, high visibility, light weight, and very thin structure. Moreover, the fast electronic response time and high luminescent efficiency associated with light-emitting organic materials allow high scan rates and low-power operation. All of these features make OLED-based displays very attractive.

5.1.3 OLED structures

A diode structure, in which the organic semiconductor is sandwiched between two electrodes, is the most commonly used scheme for LEDs (Fig. 5.1). It is speculated that the electrons in this configuration are injected into the organic material from a metal electrode (cathode), and holes are injected from the ITO electrode (anode) because ITO is n-type material. The authors think that electron extraction at the anode electrode is responsible for holes creation within organic layers. The injection of carriers from a metal into an organic material can generally be modeled by two theories: the Fowler-Nordheim (FN) model for tunnelling injection[65] and the Richardson-Schottky (RS) model for thermionic emission.[138, 148] The FN model considers the carrier injection as a process of carrier tunnelling from the metal through a triangular barrier into unbound continuum states, and ignores image charge effects that cause barrier lowering. The RS model assumes that a carrier from the metal can be injected once it has acquired enough thermal energy to surmount the potential maximum that results from the superposition of the external and the image charge potential.

Inelastic scattering of the carriers before travelling through the barrier maximum and tunnelling effects are not considered. However, in a real LED, the maximum of the electrostatic potential is located several nanometers away from the interface.[3] Ignoring this significant barrier lowering at the interface in the FN model makes it problematic. For organic light-emitting solids, the inelastic carrier scattering inside the potential well is important and cannot be ignored. This makes the application of the RS model insufficient to account for the physical process of carrier injection. Due to these deficiencies in the FN and RS models, Arkhipov et al. have come up with a theory that describes injection in similar terms as photo-conduction in organic solids. In the first step, charge and image charge pairs close to the inter-

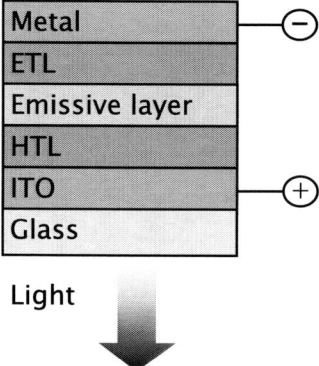

Light

Figure 5.1   Schematic of an OLED. An ITO electrode is used for hole injection, and a metal electrode is used for electron injection. The emissive organic material is separated from direct contact with the electrodes by a hole-transport layer (HTL) and an electron-transport layer (ETL).

face between the electrode and the organic are generated with the assistance of temperature and electric fields. The pair can fully dissociate in the course of a diffusive process, which is also temperature- and field-assisted. The model calculation generates results in good agreement with experimental results.[3] In order for the carriers to be efficiently injected, the contact between the electrode and the organic are made ohmic, which has a Schottky energy barrier of less than about 0.3 eV.

After the two types of carriers (electrons and holes) are created within the devices, they will drift/diffuse and recombine with each other along their diffusion pathway. The mobility of carriers plays an important role in the light-emission process. If the mobility is very low—much smaller than the 1 cm^2/Vs that is typical for organic semiconductors—the injected carriers pile up near the interface between the electrodes and the organic, and the radiative recombination rate is slow. For an optimized device, the electron and hole creation and transport should be balanced for a maximum recombination current and the highest power-conversion efficiency. A model that takes into account charge injection, transport, recombination, and space charge effects in organic materials has yielded an accurate solution for LEDs, with ohmic contacts for both electron and hole injection and high-mobility materials for balanced carrier transport.[47] In order to overcome the low carrier mobility of organic semiconductor materials, practical LED devices contain an ETL and an HTL that separate the light-emitting layer from direct contact with the electrodes. Figure 5.2 summarizes the typical internal quantum efficiency achieved by selecting electrode and carrier transport materials.[71]

Even though the emission efficiency is enhanced by incorporating electron- and hole-transport layers, other factors such as carrier injection for blue light emission are still problematic due to the large band mismatch between the electrodes and organic materials, especially for hole injection. Efficient electron injection can be achieved by choosing low work function metals, such as Ca. For electron extraction (or hole injection), one of the most suitable candidates is ITO (a high

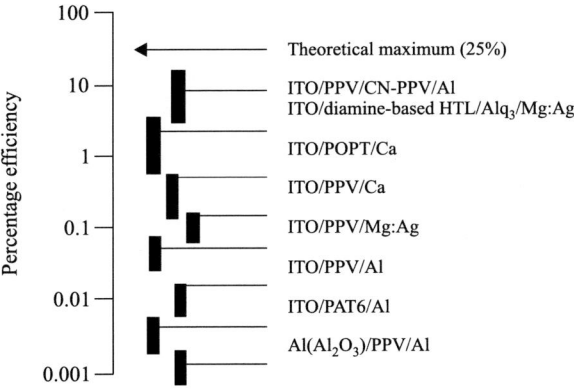

Figure 5.2 Typical internal quantum efficiencies for OLEDs. Reprinted from Ref. [70] with permission of Elsevier.

work function metal) for better light-emitting devices. However, by novel molecular-scale interface modification through self-assembly, the carrier injection efficiency of ITO can be significantly improved.

In order to grow these electro-statically self-assembled layers, solutions of polymeric ions are needed. The substrate on which the films will be grown is pre-processed to have surface charges. The substrate is alternately dipped into the polycation and the polyanion solutions to form the ionic-attracted polymer layers. Ho et al. have devised a smart design of interface layers to control carrier (especially hole) injection to achieve high EL efficiency in polymer OLEDs.[81] The goal of the ITO surface modification is to form stepped and graded electronic band profiles between the electrode and the light-emitting polymer. It turns out that partially de-doped poly(3,4-ethylenedioxythiophene): poly(4-styrenesulphonate) (PEDT:PSS) composites have different ionization energies. To fabricate the graded profile, PEDT:PSS composites are de-doped by hydrazine (N_2H_4) into different levels. The ITO surface normally contains negative charge in solution due to dangling oxygen bonds. By alternately dipping ITO substrate into polycationic poly(p-xylylene-α-tetrahydrothiophenium) (PXT) solution and polyanionic PEDT:PSS solution with various doping levels, an interface HTL forms. The final structure and schematic diagram of the band profile of the interface layer are shown in Fig. 5.3. The abrupt hole-injection (or electron-extraction) barrier between the ITO and the light-emitting polymer are graded into several smaller barrier heights, which permit a much easier carrier extraction from the light-emitting polymer. Such a scheme is expected to be especially useful for blue light-emitting polymers with large ionization energies. A green-emitting LED fabricated using this method yielded a 6% external efficiency at a luminance of 1600 cd/m^2 and at a bias of 5 V. Another approach to produce a similar effect is the insertion of the HTL between the ITO/PEDTiPSS interface and the light-emitting layer (LEL). The bandgap of HTL is larger than LEL.

There is another factor that limits the theoretical maximum internal quantum efficiency to 25%. When an organic material becomes excited through the optical energy gap, it returns to ground state by two mechanisms: fluorescence and phosphorescence. These two radiative processes share the same general mechanism but involve different excited states. A singlet state refers to a two-paired electron hole with opposite spins. A triplet state refers to a two-paired electron hole with the same spin. Fluorescence involves the transition from an excited singlet state to a singlet ground state, and phosphorescence is the transition from an excited triplet state to a singlet state.[3, 17]

In OLEDs, the injected carriers have spins, hence their means of recombination determine the spin configuration of the exciton (electron-hole pairs). Only 25% of the generated excitons are in singlet states and can emit light, while the other 75% become triplet excitons and decay through nonradiative pathways. This puts a physical limitation on the internal quantum efficiency that can be achieved in normal OLEDs. Baldo et al. have come up with a solution to harness the triplet excitons to emit light by transferring excitonic energy from a host material to a phosphorescent molecule and then to a fluorescent molecule that emits light.[17]

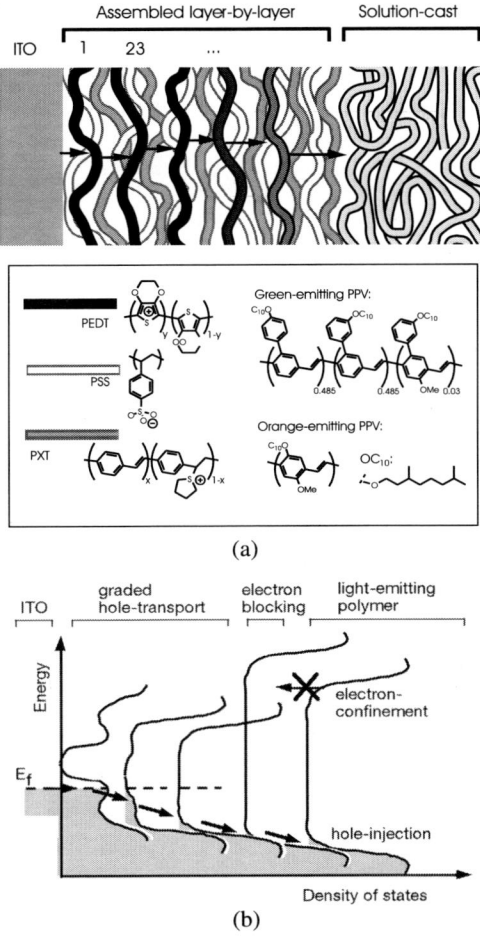

Figure 5.3 (a) Schematic of the hole-injection interlayer between the ITO electrode and the light-emitting polymer (top), and the chemical structures of the polymer (below). The interlayer consists of five graded bilayers of PEDT:PSS/PXT films plus one PSS/PXT bilayer formed by electrostatic self-assembly technique. (b) Schematic of electronic density of states across a graded interlayer. Occupied states are shaded. Holes are transported to the light-emitting material through graded lower effective barrier layers. An electron-blocking sublayer fabricated from a lower-electron-affinity polymer is also shown. Reprinted from Ref. [81] with permission of Nature/Macmillan.

There are two primary mechanisms for the energy transfer. One, called Dexter transfer, occurs over short distances and requires contact between the donor and acceptor molecules. During the transition, the exciton retains its spin configuration. Such an energy transfer is useless in terms of improving internal quantum efficiency, since triplet excitons are still forbidden to emit light. The second energy transfer pathway is called Förster transfer and can change the exciton spin configuration. This transfer does not require contact and can occur over a long distance. The different interaction ranges of the two energy transfer processes can be exploited to minimize Dexter transfer while maximizing Förster transfer. This situation can be realized by placing the phosphorescent and fluorescent molecules in alternating layers of the device. This can give an internal efficiency of fluorescence as high as 100%. The fabricated fluorescent red OLED quadruples the device efficiency. The increased efficiency reduces heating during light emission in the device and extends the lifetime of the device, since high luminance can be achieved at lower current density.

5.1.4 EL organic materials

The properties of organic light-emitting materials are different in comparison with the traditional inorganic semiconductors. Table 5.2 offers a comparison of inorganic semiconductors with polymeric light-emitting semiconductors.[71] There are two major categories of EL organic semiconductors: small molecules such as Alq$_3$, and polymers such as PPV. The two categories have in common an extended region of alternating single and double bonds in a carbon chain. In these regions, electrons form covalent bonds evenly distributed—an effect known as "conjugation." Electrons move more freely within the conjugated segments that are flat and rigid. Conjugated materials have distinctively strong coloration because these p-electrons can absorb light in the visible range. Conjugated regions can be affected by extra charge introduced to or removed from the polymer chain by chemical doping or charge injection (or extraction). Charge injection (or extraction) thus gives rise to a change in absorption as the molecule slightly rearranges itself. The color of emission is dependent on the positions of the atoms in the excited molecule, which may be different from the ground state. Some common organic light-emitting materials and their emission wavelengths are shown in Fig. 5.4.

Before the discovery of light-emitting polymers, small molecules such as 8-hydroxyquinoline Al were studied extensively for OLEDs . These materials are easy to purify and can be sublimed directly onto the device in a vacuum. Today, polymers are becoming preferred in device applications since they are expected to be more stable, particularly at high temperatures, and easier to process over large areas. There are two types of polymers used in OLEDs: precursor and soluble. Insoluble polymers, such as PPV, must be deposited in precursor form.[36] PPV precursors are soluble in methanol and water and are readily spin-coated as a thin film onto an ITO-coated substrate. Heating then converts the precursor into the fully conjugated polymer form.

The relative inertness and insolubility of the polymer make it particularly useful for multilayered devices. MEH-PPV is an example of a soluble, conjugated emissive polymer.[169] The large side-groups attached to the phenyl ring cause the polymer to be soluble in common organic solvents such as chloroform, toluene, and xylene. These bulky side-groups also make the polymer more amorphous and affect the color of the films by contributing to the conjugation of the whole molecule. Both precursor and soluble polymers offer advantages for inexpensive large-area, thin-film deposition. Some of their properties such as color, mechanical strength,

Table 5.2 Comparison of traditional and polymeric semiconductors.

Feature	Traditional Semiconductor	Polymeric Semiconductor
Band gaps	Si 1.1 eV Ge 0.67 eV GaAs 1.35 eV Relatively sharply defined	poly(acetilene) 1.4 eV PPV 2.2 eV MEH-PPV 2.1 eV Varies with polymeric segments: these are minimum band gaps
Conductivity σ Ω^{-1} cm^{-1}	Doped silicon 1 Intrinsic Si 0.0001	PPV 10^{-14} Doped poly(acetylene) max. 10^4
Doping	$<10^{20}$ cm^{-3} in crystal structure	Up to $<10^{22}$ cm^{-3} in interchain sites
Typical dopant	P, As, Sb, B (IV materials) Zn, Si (III-V materials)	I_2, AsF_5, $SbCl_5$, $FeCl_3$, O_2
Mobility μ (cm$^2V^{-1}s^{-1}$)	>1000 single crystal α-Si 0.1–10	poly(acetylene) $>10^{-3}$ PPV $<10^{-8}$
Density ρ (g cm^{-3})	Si 2.33 Ge 5.32 GaAs 5.32	PPV 1.24
Preparation	Grown from melt, sawn, and polished	Deposited from solution as thin film (polymer) or vacuum sublimed (small molecule)
Morphology	Single crystal	Disordered with tendency for molecules to lie parallel to substrate
Purity	Very high	Polymer: low Sublimed molecules: high
Transport	3D	Quasi-1D with 3D hopping to neighboring chains
Charge	Electrons and holes	Electrons and holes localized as polarons or bipolarons
Temperature dependence	$\sigma \sim e^{-\Delta\varepsilon/kT}$	$\sigma \sim e^{-A/T^{1/M}}$ (Mott hopping)
Stability	Good Diffusion of dopants High temperatures	Poor Prone to photo-oxidation Permeable to gases
Surfaces	Dangling bonds	No dangling bonds
Bulk	Covalent bonding	Molecules held by weak Van der Waals forces Atoms held covalently
Refractive index	Si 3.4 GaAs 3.6 In GaAs 3.5	PPV is anisotropic: 2.2 and 1.7

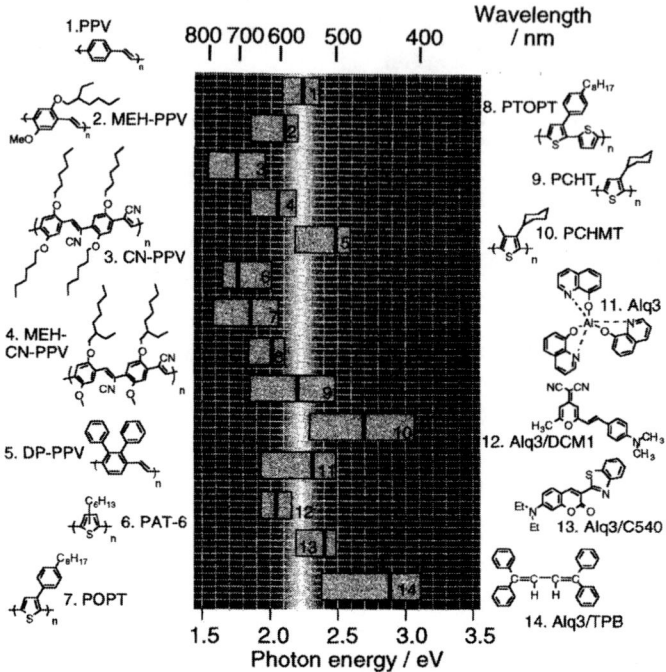

Figure 5.4 EL emission at full width, half maximum (FWHM) of a typical polymer and small-molecule light-emitting materials. Reprinted from Ref. [71] with permission of Elsevier.

and efficiency can be engineered by chemistry and processing conditions.[35] Polymer blends and copolymers with active side-chains provide a versatile way to modify properties of light-emitting polymers. Unlike PPV or MEH-PPV, which have conjugation extended along the entire polymer backbone, active segments may be incorporated into an inert polymer either in the main chain or attached as side chains.[107, 170] The material will have most of the properties of the parent polymer rather than these active segment molecules. The weakening of the EL effect due to dilution of the active segments can be balanced by an increase in quantum efficiency that arises from an increased separation between active regions.

The biggest hurdle for OLED application in consumer-grade displays lies in the potential instability of the device. Device properties may degrade in a complicated manner as a result of exposure to light, water, and oxygen molecules. The mechanisms of property degradation include the corrosion of contacts, the presence and migration of impurities, and the emissive material degradation. In most cases devices fade with time but maintain the same spectral distribution. On a microscopic level, dark spots and regions often appear, corresponding to pinholes and exposed edges of the cathode electrodes. Higher temperatures promote degradation and catastrophic failure, and are sometimes associated with local "hot spots." More details on device stability and encapsulation will be discussed later in this chapter.

5.2 Evaluation of Device Opto-Electronic Performance

Since different OLED materials and device structures affect device performance, it is necessary to characterize the OLED light output properties in order to develop high-performance OLEDs. The most common parameters that are used to describe the device performance are luminance (cd/m^2), luminous efficiency (lumen/watt), emission efficiency (cd/A), quantum efficiency, and lifetime. The brightness of OLEDs determines its application range, and the device luminous efficiency indicates the power conversion ratio and the power consumption of the device.

It is known that the emission from OLEDs is close to a Lambertian emission, especially for small angles from the normal direction to the device surface. During the evaluation of the total luminous flux of the device, it is important to have a very small surface area at the detector and a large separation between the detector and the emissive surface in order to utilize the integration of Lambertian profile to get the total luminous flux. A silicon photodiode can be used as a detector. However, a silicon photodiode cannot resolve spectra, and thus can only be used in measuring the total luminous flux and luminance of the emissive device. In order to obtain the spectral distribution of the radiant power, luminance, luminous flux, and photon emission, a calibrated spectrometer must be used. The resulting spectral curves represent the complete properties of the light emitted from the source, but also provide an accurate description of the physical properties of the device such as the EL external quantum efficiency. It is convenient to use a CCD camera to capture the spectral information of the emitted light.[75] The CCD camera needs to be carefully calibrated because the CCD's spectral response is different at different wavelengths, and this effect needs to be considered during the processing of the acquired spectral response. Once this spectral distribution of energy is obtained, the external quantum efficiency can be calculated using

$$\eta_e = \frac{N_{photon}}{N_{electron}} = \frac{\int P(\lambda)sp(\lambda)d\lambda}{J/e}, \tag{5.1}$$

where $sp(\lambda)$ is the measured spectral response from the CCD, $P(\lambda)$ is the calibration spectra of the CCD, and J is the applied current density.

5.3 Device Configuration and Display Fabrication

In this section, we discuss some of the OLED pixel and subpixel structures and fabrication processes that have high potential to be used in full-color FPDs. We begin with the basic structure of a conventional OLED and then move to more exotic pixel structures.

5.3.1 Conventional OLED

The basic structure of a conventional OLED is shown in Fig. 5.5(a). A minimum of two thin-film organic layers is required. The first layer is the HTL, and the second layer is the electron-transporting, light-emitting layer. In some cases, a third organic thin-film is used, as in Fig. 5.5(b). For this structure, the first layer is the HTL, the second thin-film is the LEL, and the third layer is the ETL. In each case, the bottom, hole-injecting (or electron-extracting) electrode is usually made of conductive ITO sputtered onto the glass substrate. The ITO electrode is transparent to visible light, and therefore, light is emitted through it when the OLED is forward-biased. The top, electron-injecting electrode (cathode) is usually a vacuum-evaporated, low work function metal or metal alloy such as Mg-Ag or Li-Al.[38] The organic layers consist of proper combinations of either small organic molecules or organic polymers. In the case of small molecules, the thin films are deposited by thermal evaporation in a vacuum. For the polymer-based OLEDs, the preferred method of deposition is spin-coating or ink-jet printing. This is a bottom light-emitting device structure. Since most of the organic materials used are sensitive to air,

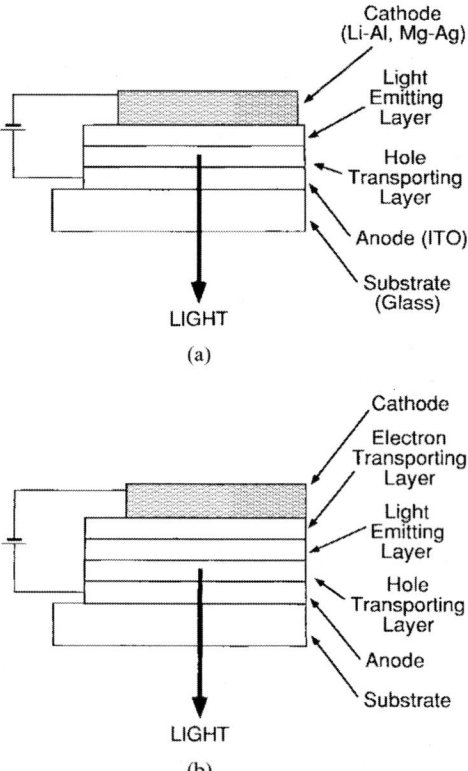

Figure 5.5 Conventional OLED structure. Reprinted from Ref. [38] with permission of the IEEE.

some form of encapsulation or passivation is usually required to reduce degradation by the formation and growth of dark-spot defects.[103]

5.3.2 Side-by-side subpixels

Figure 5.6(a) shows a side-by-side individual R, G, and B subpixel scheme, which resembles CRT arrangements. In this simple approach, each OLED subpixel requires a different light-emitting organic material. Therefore, arrays of each type of OLED must be deposited and patterned independently. This requirement may give rise to problems; for example, the patterning of one of the organic layers can cause a previous layer to swell due to the organic solvents used in the photolithographic processes, or to deteriorate due to the relatively high processing temperatures used in the etching process.[38] However, by using the side-by-side pixel scheme, 300-dpi displays have been fabricated.[38]

Some fabrication techniques can be used to overcome these limitations. One technique, described by Burrows et al.,[38] uses dielectric "walls" that have been patterned on the substrate to separate each subpixel and to shadow two of the three subpixels from the unwanted thermal deposition of the light-emitting material. By tilting the substrate for each of the three organic layer growths, R, G, and B organic material can be grown in separate areas, thereby providing three distinct subpixels. However, nonuniformity can result from the difficulties of controlling the deposition area. Another technique is the precision shadow-mask method. In this approach, selective deposition of R, G, and B organic materials is done with a thin mask and a high-accuracy mask-moving mechanism. To obtain good patterning and better size control, the mask should be thin and the distance between the mask and the substrate should be as small as possible. Unfortunately, due to the thin mask requirement, difficulties arise because the mask must be kept flat, which leads to a nonuniform gap between the mask and the substrate. This is especially true for large-area substrates. In the side-by-side subpixel technique, the light emission from each subpixel is controlled independently and can be optimized separately to reach higher quantum and power efficiency. In summary, the unevenness of the mask, nonuniform gaps, and nonuniformity caused by oblique deposition hinder this technique from its use for large-area display fabrication.

5.3.3 White OLED filtering

Figure 5.6(b) presents another pixel scheme that can be used to realize a full-color display. This color subtraction scheme can be compared to LCDs in that the white OLED serves as a "backlight" and the emitted light is passed through separate R, G, and B filters. The white OLED is fabricated by deposition of two or more organic layers that emit different colors (R, G, and B) onto a prepatterned substrate. The thickness of each organic layer is such that the superposition of the light emit-

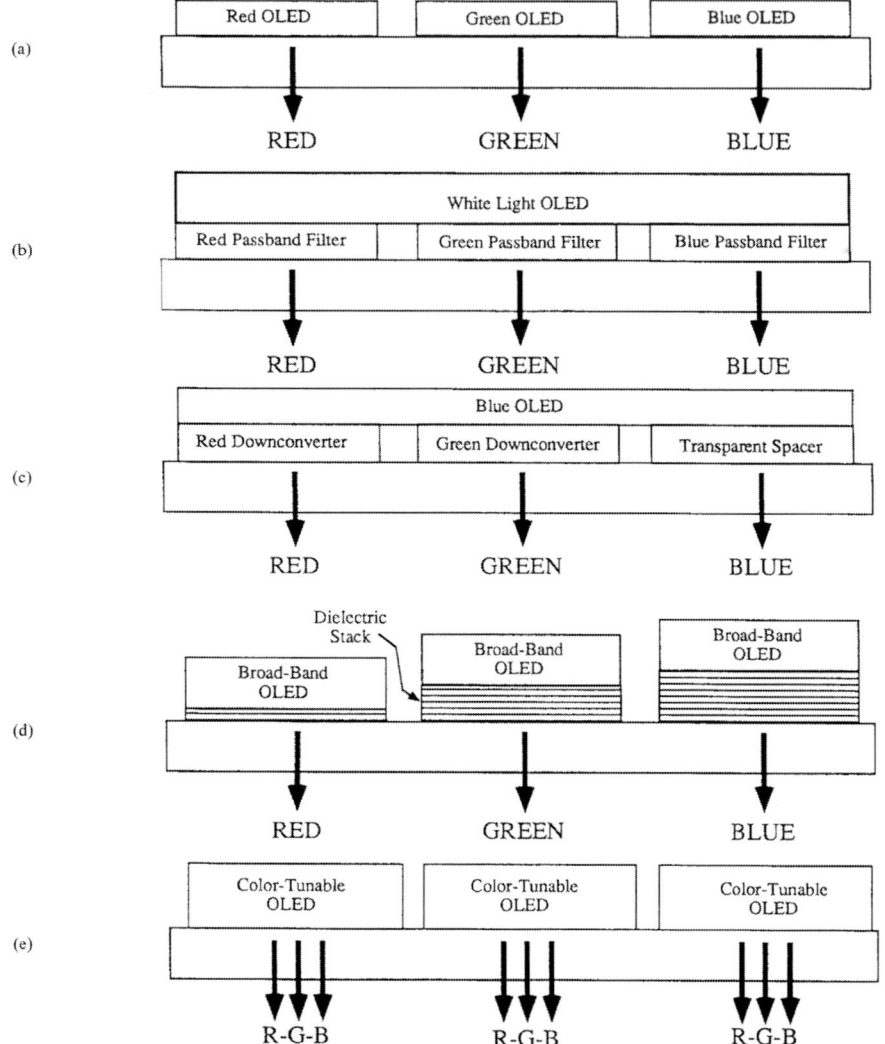

Figure 5.6   Five full-color subpixel configurations. Reprinted from Ref. [38] with permission of the IEEE.

ted appears white. No post-deposition patterning is required since only one white OLED structure is grown over the entire substrate.[70] However, this pixel design approach has limitations. The main disadvantage is that most of the emitted light (up to 90% of the optical power) is absorbed by the filter to achieve a fully saturated color subpixel. This requires the OLED to be driven at a higher current density to achieve sufficient brightness. Unfortunately, a high current density produces more defects and heat, and accelerates OLED degradation.[38] Even with these limitations, white OLED filtering is still a viable technique that can be used in the fabrication of FPDs where power consumption is not a major concern, but good device stability is required.

5.3.4 Blue OLED down-conversion

Figure 5.6(c) illustrates a photoluminescent method to realize separate R, G, and B subpixels. A blue OLED is used to optically pump a prepatterned subpixel, which consists of a fluorescent material that absorbs the blue light and emits either red or green light. For blue light, a transparent layer (spacer) is used in place of the red or green fluorescent organic material. Even though the power efficiency of this system can be low because the energy of the emitted red or green photon is less than the energy of the absorbed blue photon, the conversion quantum efficiency (photons out/photons in) can be near 100%.[38]

A major problem with this technique is the guiding of light, by the substrate, into the neighboring subpixels, causing unwanted photoluminescence. This is a form of optical crosstalk and causes color bleeding in the subpixels, which reduces the contrast of the display. Burrows et al. have demonstrated that the substrate guiding of the light, and therefore the color bleeding, can be reduced by using a shaped substrate that enhances forward light scattering.[38] For example, the structure shown in Fig. 5.7(b) greatly improves the output coupling of light, as compared to the structure in Fig. 5.7(a).

5.3.5 Microcavity OLEDs

Figure 5.6(d) shows the use of microcavity filters to realize R, G, and B subpixels based on an inherently broadband OLED. Microcavities have been shown to be an effective method to control the direction and color of OLED emissions. The microcavity is formed by the reflective metal electrode on the top of the OLED and a dielectric, quarter-wavelength, multilayer structure that has been fabricated under the transparent ITO in the bottom of the structure. When a white OLED is placed in this cavity, the OLED will emit light of a certain color in a certain direction.[38] In this approach, the emission's spectral bandwidth becomes narrower and the intensity is enhanced due to the microcavity effect. Under careful design (i.e., changing the length of the cavity), it is possible to position the emission in the desired wavelength band. The increase of emission intensity reduces the required driving current, thereby reducing power consumption. Thus, degradation of OLEDs is reduced and lifetime increases.

This technique does have two main limitations. The first is the directional dependence of the wavelength selection. In other words, different colors are preferentially seen at different angles from the microcavity OLED structure. Typically, the viewing angle is around 15 deg for a 10:1 luminance decrease. Secondly, the different microcavity structures for R, G, and B create a wide variation in thickness, and this thickness is usually larger than the organic layer. Therefore, it is difficult to deposit a continuous, high-quality organic light-emitting layer on the substrate containing the prepatterned microcavity structures.[38] Microcavities are, however, an important means of tuning the color of the emitted light.

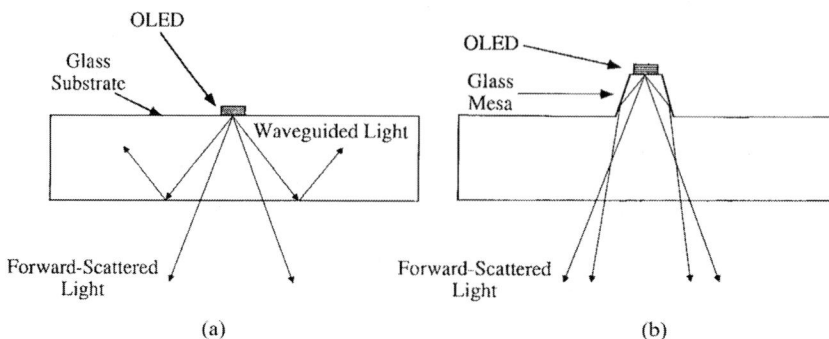

Figure 5.7 Schematic cross-section of an OLED grown on (a) a plain substrate, and (b) a mesa-shaped substrate. Reprinted from Ref. [38] with permission of the IEEE.

5.3.6 Color-tunable OLEDs

Figure 5.6(e) illustrates the concept of using a single, color-tunable OLED. This scheme eliminates the need for individual R, G, and B subpixels to create one full-color pixel, which results in an enhancement of the display resolution and pixel fill factor by a factor of three compared to previously discussed pixel schemes.[63] Due to the fact that only one OLED configuration is grown over the entire surface, the need for prepatterning the substrate is removed, thereby providing a simpler fabrication process. However, this advantage trades off with the requirement of more complex driving circuits, because the circuit must be able to control simultaneously the color, brightness, and gray level of the OLED. One method that has been used to achieve a color-tunable OLED involves a polymer blend or polymer electrochemical cell as the light-emitting organic material. Each ingredient of the blend or cell emits at a different wavelength. The color and brightness (gray level) can be tuned by applying different voltages and/or a different polarity to the OLED, i.e., high voltage pushes the emitted color into the blue region and lower voltage corresponds to more red light emission. However, the higher voltage also causes higher current injection, and therefore affects the brightness of the OLED.[38] This method also has problems achieving full color due to the ever-present lower energy light emission regions and possible accelerated degradation of the OLED at high current levels.

5.3.7 Pyramid-shaped pixel OLEDs

The idea of using pyramid-shaped pixel OLEDs to achieve color has been published recently.[168] In this technique, different organic materials, emitting different colors, are deposited on each surface of a pyramid-shaped structure. The basic concept is similar to that of side-by-side subpixels, but this approach provides a three-fold enhancement in the resolution because three subpixels are integrated

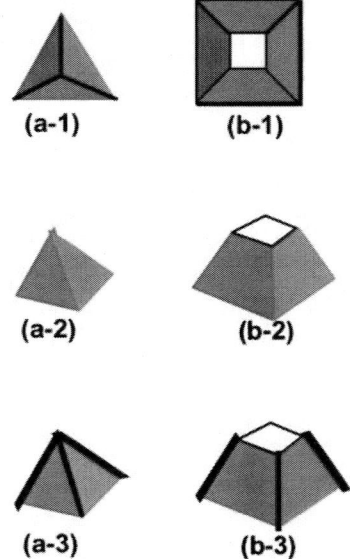

Figure 5.8 Different structures of pyramid-shaped pixels. Diagrams (a-3) and (b-3) show the dielectric mask wall. Reprinted from Ref. [168] with permission of the American Institute of Physics.

into one pixel. The fabrication processes seem to be relatively easy and require oblique thermal deposition of organic materials. As different materials are deposited, only a rotation of the samples is needed. Thus, this process requires no mask. The different pyramid structures that can be used are shown in Fig. 5.8. To guarantee that proper materials are deposited on the correct surfaces, a dielectric mask wall on the edges is fabricated before evaporation, which provides better shielding. In addition to the aforementioned advantages, the pyramid-shaped structure also largely enhances the extraction quantum efficiency and reduces the optical waveguiding effect. A demonstration by use of an optical prism to simulate a pyramid-shaped structure is shown in Fig. 5.9.

Although this technique has many advantages, pyramid-shaped substrates are needed, which complicates the fabrication process and increases cost. Furthermore, due to the pyramid shapes, the viewing angle is limited. At least one color is blocked by pyramid structures at large off-axis viewing angles. The electrical connections and addressing scheme are also challenging. A more promising method to implement a color-tunable device is the stacked OLED.[64]

5.3.8 Stacked OLEDs

Stacked OLEDs (SOLEDs) have the potential to provide the highest image resolution simultaneously with low fabrication costs. As depicted in Fig. 5.10, the SOLED consists of a stacked blue OLED, green OLED, and red OLED. Most organic mol-

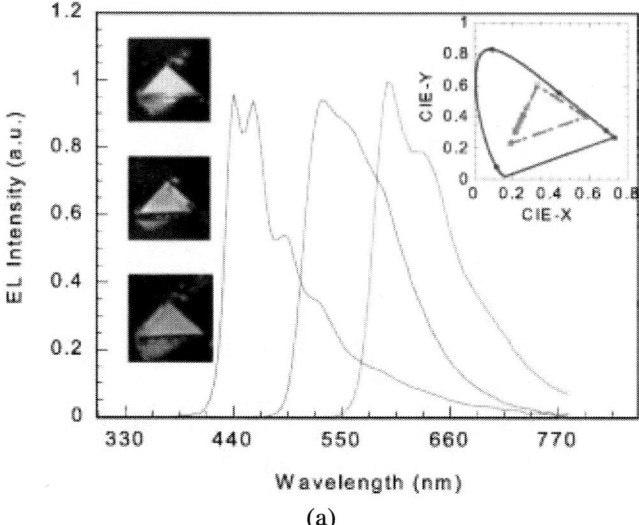

(a)

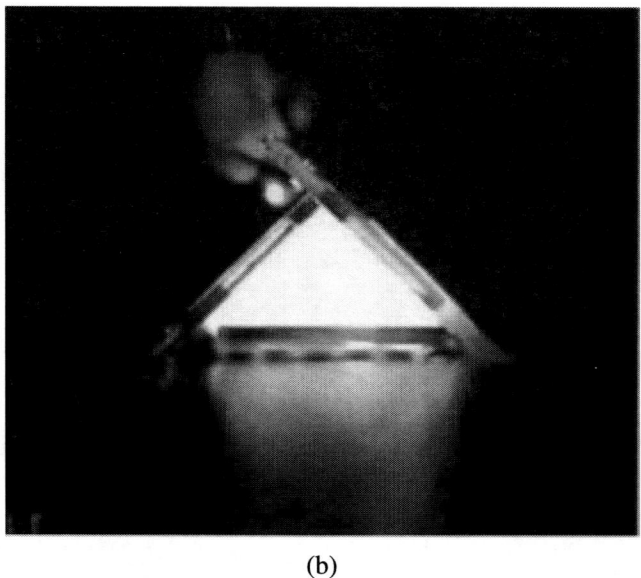

(b)

Figure 5.9 (a) Measured spectra of R, G, and B elements. (b) Picture shows white light emission as R, G, and B are turned on simultaneously. Reprinted from Ref. [168] with permission of the American Institute of Physics.

ecules and polymers on which these OLEDs are based have an emission spectrum that is red-shifted from the absorption spectrum. This property causes OLEDs to be transparent to their own emitted light and to most of the spectrum of visible light, giving rise to the transparent OLED (TOLED). Therefore, TOLEDs can be stacked on top of each other with only a small reduction in efficiency.

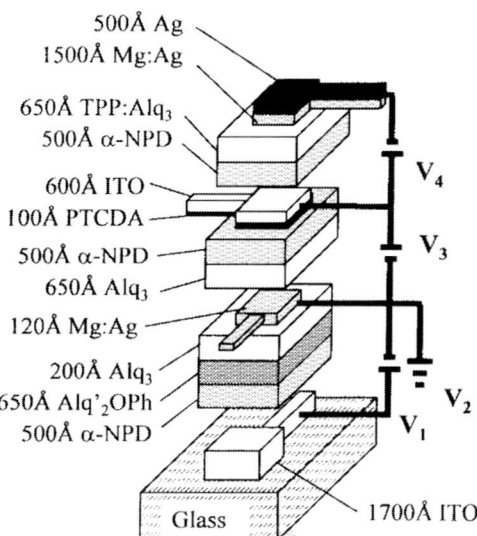

500Å Ag
1500Å Mg:Ag
650Å TPP:Alq$_3$
500Å α-NPD
600Å ITO
100Å PTCDA
500Å α-NPD
650Å Alq$_3$
120Å Mg:Ag
200Å Alq$_3$
650Å Alq'$_2$OPh
500Å α-NPD
V_4
V_3
V_2
V_1
Glass
1700Å ITO

Figure 5.10 Stacked OLED (SOLED). Reprinted from Ref. [38] with permission of the IEEE.

The fabrication process to form this structure is relatively simple and does not involve etching of the organic materials. A transparent ITO layer is deposited on a glass substrate. This ITO functions as the anode to the blue OLED. The blue OLED is formed by the successive deposition of an HTL, a blue LEL, and then an ETL. A thin (~ 100 Å) and approximately 50% transparent Mg-Ag alloy is thermally evaporated onto the structure to serve as the cathode for both the blue and green OLEDs. To form the inverted green OLED, a green, fluorescent, organic thin-film is deposited. Next, an HTL is added, followed by the sputtering of ITO to form the shared anode for the green and red OLEDs. To form the red OLED, a third HTL is deposited. Then a red LEL is deposited followed by the deposition of a thick (~ 1500 Å) Mg-Ag electron-injecting cathode. To finish the structure, a layer of Ag is deposited to reduce oxidation of the Mg.[38] A structure of this nature can only be achieved with the use of organic materials; no such structure, constructed from numerous heterogeneous layers, could be fabricated using crystalline inorganic materials due to their strict lattice-matching requirements.

A useful variation of the SOLED structure can be formed by splitting the top ITO electrode (i.e., the electrode shared by the green and red OLEDs) into two separate electrodes. This can be easily achieved by depositing a transparent insulating oxide or organic layer following the ITO deposition. Then another layer of ITO can be deposited to form the anode of the red OLED. This structure is slightly more complex, but has several advantages. One significant advantage is the simplification of the driving circuit. The previous SOLED structure, with the shared ITO electrode, necessitates differential biasing of the red OLED and therefore requires a complex driving scheme. With the splitting of the electrode, each OLED can be addressed independently, and the driving circuit is similar to the one used by the lateral subpixel scheme. Another advantage of this structure is the use of the thickness of the transparent insulating layer to tune the optical cavity length, thereby eliminating or reducing unwanted microcavity effects.[64] The final SOLED structure is three separate, stacked R, G, and B subpixels that can be addressed independently, providing one full-color pixel.

In the SOLED structure, some drawbacks are inevitable. Semitransparent electrodes for the middle subpixel introduce a loss of efficiency due to light absorption. Fortunately, several low-absorption metal-containing or metal-free electrodes, such as CuPc and BCP, have been found to reduce absorption and enhance the efficiency.[70] Additionally, these electrodes are able to reduce the microcavity effects. Another problem is color bleeding due to energy down-conversion of light emitted from the blue OLED upon passing through the red LEL. This problem can be minimized by the use of guest-host doped layers for the devices emitting at longer wavelengths.

To sum up all the subpixel techniques we have discussed, a review of the main advantages and disadvantages of each structure is presented in Table 5.3.

5.4 OLED Stability and Encapsulation for Displays

In this section, the detrimental impact of moisture and oxygen on OLED properties is addressed with a description of the formation, growth, and influence of dark spots. Then, several methods to encapsulate OLEDs are briefly summarized.

5.4.1 Impact of moisture and oxygen

Even though the good performance of OLEDs in inert gases has been demonstrated, the lifetime in air is very short and therefore inadequate for commercial applications. The short lifetime of an OLED is due to its exposure to water vapor and oxygen that are present in the air.[28, 68] A basic OLED is composed of a transparent electrode such as ITO, an EL layer, and a metal layer. The influences of air exposure on each layer are described in detail below.

The polymers used in the EL layer are usually very sensitive to photo-oxidation. This leads to an interruption of the polymer conjugation length by changing their chemical structures. A reduction of conjugation length and polymer bleaching will be the final result of this process. To verify this process experimentally, a Kr laser with the wavelength at 482 nm was used to irradiate PPV, which is typically used as the EL layer, and the transmission was measured as a function of time under three different conditions. According to the results, shown in Fig. 5.11, the increase of PPV's transmission with exposure time in air is more rapid than that occurring in water vapor and a vacuum. Hence, water vapor was able to cause photobleaching, e.g., an increase of polymer transmission; so was oxygen. Moreover, the influence of oxygen on the polymer degradation was stronger than that of water vapor.

Table 5.3 Summary of different subpixel structures used to achieve full-color displays.

Technique	Advantages	Disadvantages
Side-by-side RGB (shadow-mask method)	1. No power penalty 2. High quantum and power efficiency 3. Low fabrication cost	1. Low resolution 2. Limited display panel size
Filtering of white OLED by absorptive filters	1. High resolution 2. Easy fabrication 3. Can be transplanted from LCD technology	1. Low efficiency 2. High driving current 3. Short lifetime 4. High power consumption 5. Expensive color filters
Filtering of white OLED by dielectric multilayer structure	1. Enhanced output intensity 2. Slightly lower driving current	1. Complex fabrication 2. Small viewing angle
Down-conversion of blue light to red and green light	1. High resolution	1. Low contrast 2. High fabrication cost 3. Color bleeding
Color-tunable pixels	1. High resolution 2. Tunable spectrum	1. High operating voltage 2. Fast degradation 3. Complex drivers
Pyramid-shaped pixels	1. High resolution 2. Mask-free fabrication 3. Enhanced quantum efficiency	1. Pyramid-shaped substrates needed 2. Small viewing angle 3. Complicated electrical connections and addressing scheme
Stacked OLED (SOLED)	1. High resolution 2. High efficiency	1. Absorption by semitransparent electrode 2. Color bleeding 3. Microcavity effect 4. Complex drivers

The cathode in OLEDs is used to inject electrons into the EL layer. It should be made of a metal with a low work function. However, if it is exposed to water vapor or oxygen, it will very quickly form metal oxide due to its highly reactive nature. Instead of direct metal corrosion, water vapor and oxygen can also permeate through the cathode and form oxide at the interface between the metal and polymer layers. This was also verified by the measurement of x-ray photon-electron spectroscopy (XPS). The XPS spectrum is shown in Fig. 5.12. The oxide layer present at the metal interface polymer has negative effects on the device's performance since it modifies the barrier for electron injection into the EL layer. A higher resistance present at this interface will require a large current density or voltage value to produce light emission.

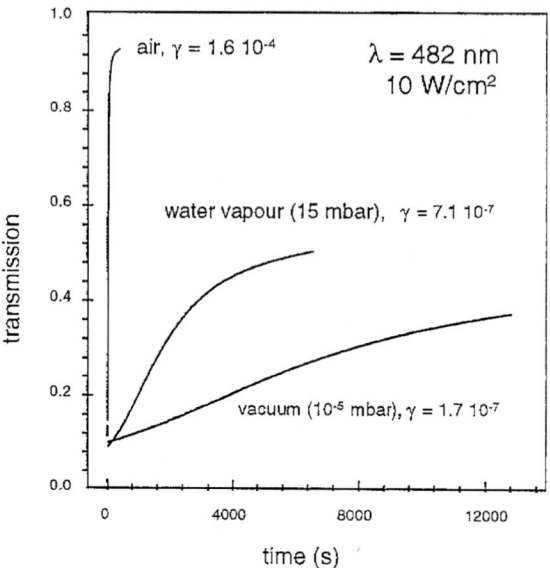

Figure 5.11 Evolution of PPV transmission under air, water vapor, and a vacuum with time exposure. Adapted from Ref. [28] with permission of Elsevier.

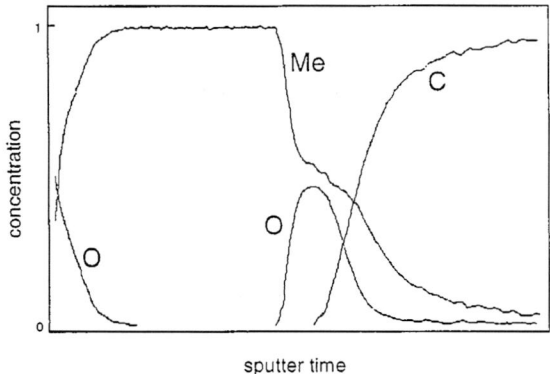

Figure 5.12 XPS spectrum of an OLED. Adapted from Ref. [28] with permission of Elsevier.

The anode in an OLED is used to extract electrons from (or inject holes into) the EL layer. Although there are papers[28, 29] reporting that a UV/ozone or oxygen plasma treatment of ITO can improve OLED performance considerably, the improvements are not stable. This treatment will increase oxygen concentration at the ITO surface. Since oxygen is electro-negative, it will form a negatively charged surface layer at the ITO/EL layer interface resulting in repulsion and depletion of electrons just beneath the surface of the ITO. This will induce band bending and a higher work function of the ITO that is responsible for a higher density of holes near the interface.

5.4.2 Influence of dark spots

Another fatal factor that can greatly reduce an OLED's lifetime is dark spot formation. There are at least two possible origins of dark spots. One is due to dust particles,[111, 117] and the other is due to high local-current flux.[66]

Dust is unavoidable in the OLED fabrication processes. Dust particles create a shadow effect during evaporation of the organic material and leave spaces inside the light-emitting material. If the dimension of the particles is larger than the thickness of the OLEDs, there is no doubt that the device will not emit light from this region. Moreover, water and oxygen can more easily penetrate into the devices through these large areas, because even if the dust particle size is smaller than the OLED thickness, they provide sufficient spaces for water and oxygen to permeate inside the film. Figure 5.13 shows the time evolution of dark spots. It should be noted that the size of dark spots increases with time but their number typically remains the same.

The high local-current density is another cause of dark spots. From the EL measurement it was concluded that bright spots will evolve into dark spots, which can be seen in Fig. 5.14. The bright spots probably come from a high local conductivity due to the reduced thickness of the EL layer, a thicker metal film, or better contacts. As soon as bright spots are formed, the local-current density becomes very high, which will cause a local increase in temperature due to large local joule heating. Unfortunately, the higher the temperature, the larger the polymer's conductivity, resulting in positive feedback. The high temperature can also trigger the interdiffusion of organic layers and/or contact metal inside the OLED layer, which will result in a low conductivity and the formation of dark spots. As time goes by, the size of the dark spots grows. The stages of this effect are shown in Fig. 5.15.

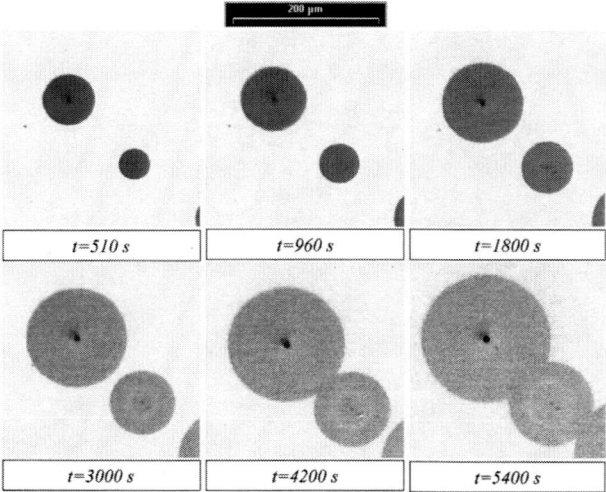

Figure 5.13 Time evolution of dark spot formation. Reprinted from Ref. [111] with permission of the American Institute of Physics.

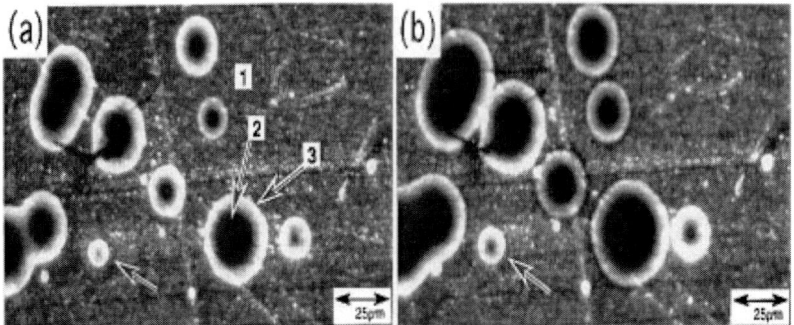

Figure 5.14 EL spectra showing dark and bright spots at different stages of formation. Reprinted from Ref. [66] with permission of the American Institute of Physics.

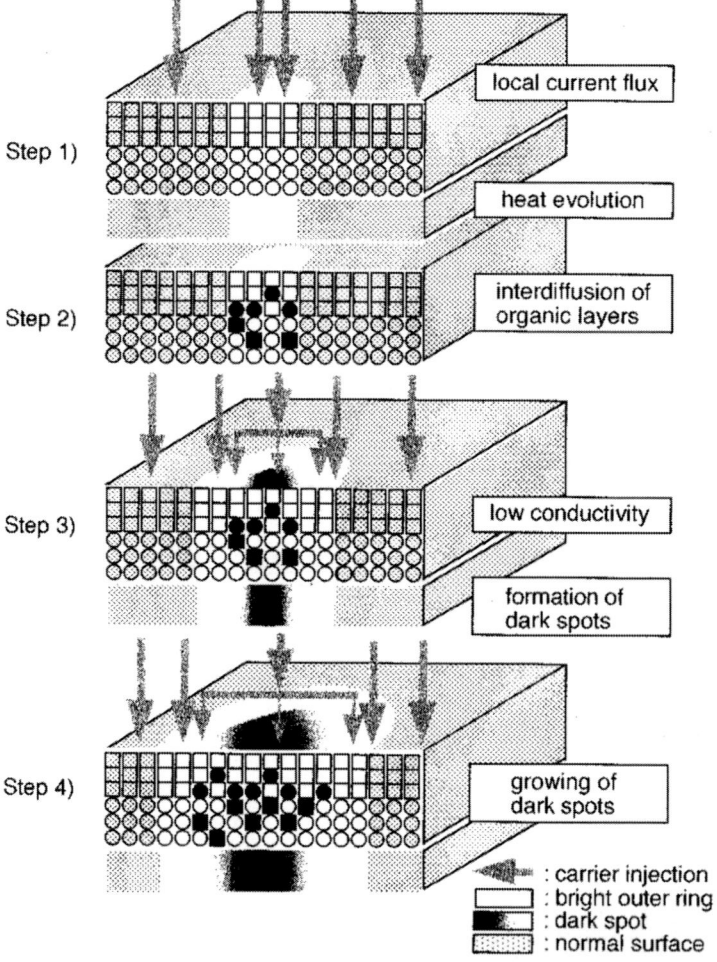

Figure 5.15 A propagation mechanism of dark spots. Reprinted from Ref. [66] with permission of the American Institute of Physics.

These dark spots are related more to the nonuniform OLED structure than to the influence of vapor and oxygen.

5.4.3 Encapsulation methods

To solve the problem of OLED lifetime, several methods have been proposed to encapsulate and seal OLEDs from humidity and oxygen. The simplest way is to use glass as a top cap with a nitrogen-filled chamber.[37] A schematic of the structure is shown in Fig. 5.16. This configuration uses epoxy, a widely used encapsulant in electronic packaging. In addition, a-SiN$_x$ is deposited to reduce the permeability of humidity and oxygen from the sides.

Another method is to encapsulate OLEDs by sealing canisters with a UV adhesive such as epoxy resin under a nitrogen atmosphere,[103] which is a common method to seal semiconductor LEDs. In addition, a plasma-enhanced chemical vapor deposition (PECVD) silicon nitride film (a-SiN$_x$) is always deposited for passivation to provide low film stress and a good barrier against humidity and oxygen, with BaO added as a resistive absorbent.

The third approach utilizes a stack of alternating polymer and transparent dielectric layers to protect OLEDs from the permeation of water and oxygen through the substrate.[73] Preferably, the dielectric layer is fabricated from silicon monoxide (SiO), silicon oxide (SiOx), silicon dioxide (SiO$_2$), or silicon nitride (Si$_3$N$_4$). As for the polymer layer, it can be chosen from a group of robust polymers such as fluorinated polymers, parylenes, and cyclotenes. On top of the OLEDs, the hermetic sealing consists of several layers including a buffer layer, followed by a thermal coefficient matching layer, and then an inorganic layer with low permeability. The buffer layer may be either an organic polymer, such as a parylene with

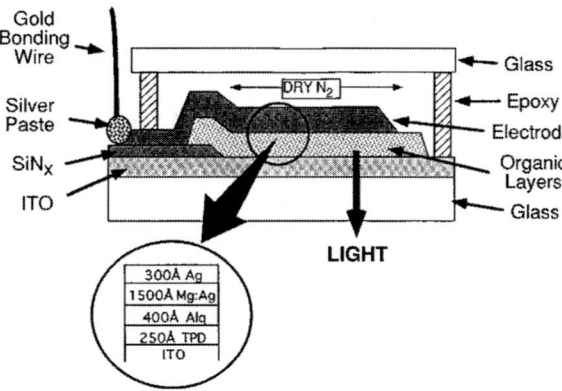

Figure 5.16 Schematic cross-section of an encapsulated, nitrogen-filled OLED with a detailed view of the thin-film layers. Reprinted from Ref. [37] with permission of the American Institute of Physics.

a low thermal expansion coefficient, or an organometallic complex such as Alq_3. For example, SiO_2 can be used as the thermal coefficient matching layer while Si_3N_4 functions as the inorganic outermost layer. A schematic side view is shown in Fig. 5.17. Outside the plurality of layers, epoxy and a thin metal foil can be added to strengthen its effectiveness against water and oxygen permeation.

The fourth approach[141] is similar to the first one. It uses glass, quartz, or thin silicon as a cap to provide cost and weight advantages. The perimetric seal is comprised of an electrically insulating layer, adhesion layers, and sealing layers, which is depicted in Fig. 5.18. Usually indium, tin, or gold is used for the sealing layers and titanium is used as the adhesion layers. The sealing process is accomplished by using pressure and a heating element.

The last method does not use epoxy coating, which tends to degrade the device property due to the infiltration of the solvent into the EL layer. In this scheme, a dielectric layer is coated on top of metallic cathodes and a metal film is added above the dielectric layer.[91] The basic structure is shown in Fig. 5.19. Although the polymers used to protect devices in some approaches have excellent electrical resistivity, the high breakdown strength and transparency, and the ability to avoid permeation of water, are not good enough. Furthermore, some metal films

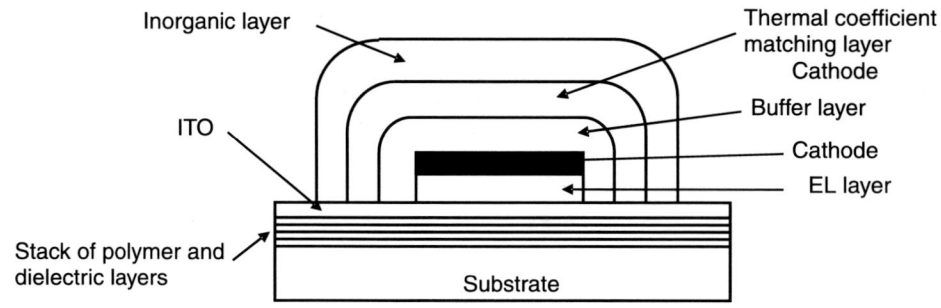

Figure 5.17   Cross-section side view of an encapsulated OLED.

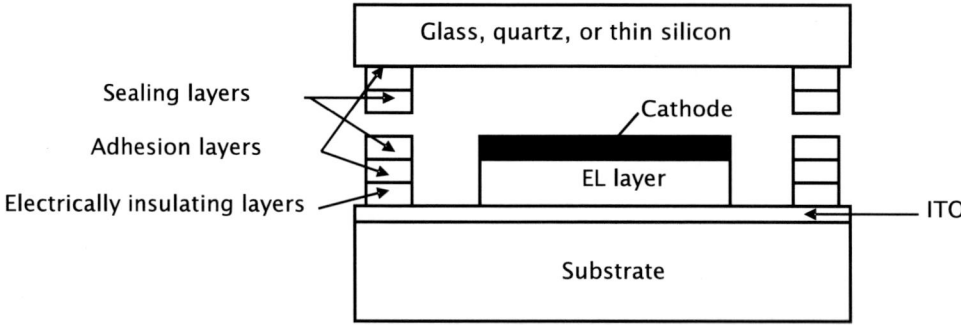

Figure 5.18   Side view of an encapsulated OLED.

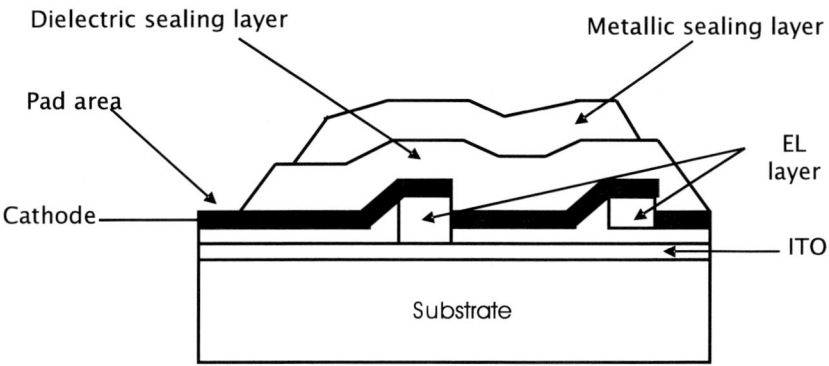

Figure 5.19 Cross section of an encapsulated OLED. Adapted from Ref. [170] with permission of Elsevier.

are also used to seal OLEDs, but they should be relatively thick to avoid pinholes, which leads to poor light transmission. In this method, only two thin layers are needed. The dielectric layer is preferably composed of a SiC film with a thickness of 500 nm, deposited by PECVD from trimethylsilane. Alternatively, diamond-like carbon (DLC), SiO, SiO_2, Si_3N_4, or silicon oxynitride (SiO_xN_y) can also be used. The PECVD-deposited SiC provides high dielectric strength, good film adhesion, a low pinhole density, and impermeability. Additionally, this dielectric layer may consist of a combination of several materials—for example, SiO_2 and SiC, DLC and SiC, or Si_3N_4 and SiO_2. As for the metal film, it is better to use sputtering deposition. Sometimes, a combination of PECVD and an electron beam or sputtering deposition achieves the lowest pinhole density. The function of the metal film is to reduce the device's susceptibility to cracking under stress, and to preseal the pinholes. The device is then baked, preferably in purified air or a dry nitrogen-oxygen atmosphere. The metals will react with oxygen or moisture to adsorb gases and seal off pinholes inside the layer. This beneficial property removes pathways for oxygen and moisture. When patterning the dielectric and metal films, a shadow mask may be employed where external connections are required.

5.5 Display Addressing and Driving Circuit

In this section, we describe several addressing schemes and driving circuits that have been used to control OLED flat-panel devices. We assume that the data timing and multiplexing to the appropriate column electrode has been taken care of so we can focus on the individual pixel driving mechanisms. Two main categories of display driving schemes exist: direct addressing and matrix addressing. We will begin with a short description of direct addressing and then move to the explanation of two different types of matrix addressing.

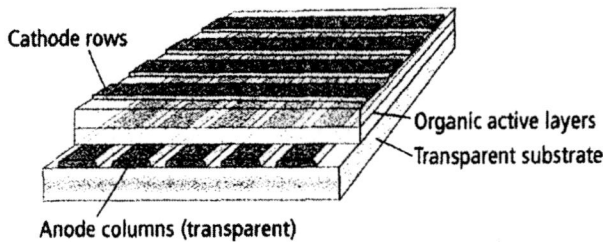

Figure 5.20 Matrix addressing of an OLED. Adapted from Ref. [64] with permission of the IEEE.

In direct addressing, each pixel is connected to an individual driver. This scheme is most efficiently used in alphanumeric displays, such as the common seven-segment display, and discrete indicator displays.[70] This type of addressing is not applicable to video-rate FPD technology. However, direct addressing is useful where the display is relatively simple and low-information contents are displayed, but the pixel is in the form of a complex pattern that is simply turned on and off.

In matrix addressing, the pixels are arranged into a two-dimensional array of rows and columns. Each pixel is then connected to one row lead and one column lead as shown in Fig. 5.20.[64] The matrix addressing scheme in which active electronic devices such as TFTs are used to enhance the display characteristics is termed active-matrix (AM) addressing. A much simpler addressing scheme in which no extra active electronic devices are used is termed passive-matrix (PM) addressing. With the use of matrix addressing schemes, arrays of OLEDs can be used as high information content and video-rate FPDs.[70]

5.5.1 PM-addressing method

In a PM-addressed display, the organic light emitter is connected to a row electrode and an orthogonal, electrically isolated, column electrode. An equivalent circuit of this scheme is shown in Fig. 5.21. The diode represents the OLED sandwiched at the intersection of the row and column electrodes. The fabrication process is relatively simple. First, the row electrode (anode) material, usually ITO, is deposited onto the transparent glass substrate and then patterned using photolithography to achieve fine features. Next, the organic layers are deposited in one of the schemes discussed above to create R, G, and B subpixels. Finally, the conducting column electrode material (metal alloy cathode) is deposited using a shadow mask to avoid the exposure of the organic layers to moisture during the etching of the electrode lines. The mechanical shadow mask method does not give nearly the resolution that is provided by photolithography.

The operation principle of a PM-addressed display is straightforward. Each row electrode (anode) is connected to an electronic switch and each column elec-

Column Electrodes

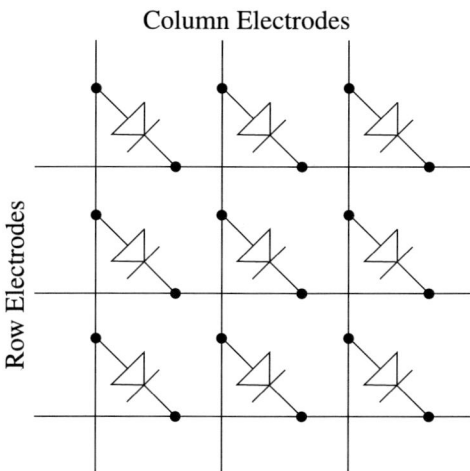

Figure 5.21 Equivalent circuit of the PM-addressing scheme.

trode (cathode) is connected to a current source. Since light emission from the pixel is dependent on the current passing through the OLED, current sources must be used to effectively realize different gray levels.[70] The row electrodes are scanned in succession (row-by-row) at a frame rate that is greater than 60 frames per second. The data signals, which are electric current signals, are applied to the column electrodes with the proper timing, thereby successively turning the pixels on and off.

Several disadvantages exist with the PM-addressing scheme. One problem is caused when one of the pixels in the display malfunctions, i.e., the pixel is shorted or leaky. This can cause other pixels near the "bad" pixel to be unintentionally addressed. This event is one of many forms of crosstalk and disrupts the normal operation of the display. Another problem is due to an inherent characteristic of the OLED. Consider a display with M rows. With the row-by-row scanning scheme, each of the OLEDs is powered on for a maximum of $1/M$ of the frame period. Since OLEDs have no memory effect, they will be off unless they are addressed and driven by the external power source. In order to achieve the required average display panel brightness of, for example, 100 cd/m^2 in a frame period, each OLED must be driven at a brightness of $M \times 100$ cd/m^2. Large currents are needed to achieve the required brightness when M is large, thereby causing accelerated degradation of the OLED. Besides, the OLED emission efficiency decreases at a high current level, which also causes fast degradation of the OLED. Another disadvantage arises from the number and size of electrode lines used in the display. If M is large, appreciable and unwanted voltage drops may occur across the electrodes, causing the pixels to display incorrect information. This limits the total number of rows to approximately 500, which is far below the number required for a high-information content and a high-resolution FPD.[70] AM-addressing schemes can be used to alleviate these problems.

5.5.2 AM-addressing method

As stated above, matrix addressing schemes that utilize active electronic components at each pixel site are termed active matrix (AM). These active switching elements are usually TFTs with poly-Si, a-Si:H, or an organic semiconducting small molecule or polymer film (OTFTs) used as the channel region material. Due to the lack of memory effect in OLEDs, at least two TFTs per pixel (or subpixel for full-color displays) are needed for an effective AM-addressing circuit (see Fig. 5.22).

The circuit has one control line (V_{select}), one data line (V_{data}), and power/ground lines. The external driving circuits consist of gate and source drivers. The V_{select} line is connected to the gate drivers, and the source drivers supply data to the source of T1 in each pixel circuit. The V_{select} line is set to high for data to be written to the pixel. Here, the signal V_{data} charges the storage capacitor to the desired voltage (C_{st}). The voltage on the storage capacitor remains constant even after V_{select} switches to low (–5 V) except for the initial drop due to the parasitic capacitance of T1 when T1 turns off. The current flowing through the OLED (I_{OLED}) is controlled by the drive transistor, T2. When T2 is biased in saturation, the current I_{OLED} is

$$I_{OLED} = \frac{\mu C W}{2L}(V_{GS} - V_{th})^2, \qquad (5.2)$$

where μ, C, W, and L are the channel mobility, the channel capacitance, the channel width, and the channel length of the transistor, respectively; V_{GS} is the gate to the source voltage; and V_{th} is the threshold voltage of the TFT.

In the voltage driving configuration, a slight threshold voltage variation in the OLED could be the result of the long-term operation or the process nonuniformity. This variation will charge the current flowing through the OLED since the V_{GS} of T2 is dependent on the drop across the OLED. When a current driving circuit is used and V_{DD} is large (T2 in deep saturation), the variation in threshold

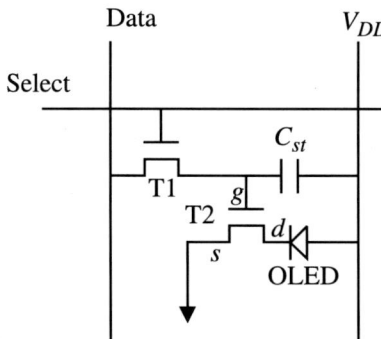

Figure 5.22 AM-addressing scheme using two TFTs per pixel.

voltage of the OLED will not affect the current because the V_{GS} of T2 remains unchanged. Therefore, a constant current configuration circuit is preferred for an AMOLED. This type of OLED addressing will be discussed in more detail below.

5.6 TFT Technology for AM Displays

The TFT is an important switching and driving element in the AM-addressing scheme. The TFT is also an essential element for achieving high-resolution and integrated-driver AM addressing. The TFTs can be made using a-Si:H, poly-Si, or organic semiconductors as the active region of the TFT. Although we will not go into the details of the electrical properties of these devices, we will present two requirements that must be fulfilled in order for the TFTs to be effective in the pixel electrode driving circuits that are discussed below. For the details, the reader is referred to Ref. [70]. In order to fully charge the storage capacitor of the pixel circuit, the ON-current must be sufficiently large. Also, in order to maintain the bias on the gate of T2, the OFF-current must be sufficiently small. This leads to the first TFT requirement, which is the ON-current (I_{on}) to OFF-current (I_{off}) ratio

$$\frac{I_{on}}{I_{off}} \geq 2SMN_g .\tag{5.3}$$

Here, S is an engineering safety margin, M is the number of rows, and N_g is the number of gray levels. If we take $M = 1024$, $N_g = 256$, and $S = 3$, then $I_{on}/I_{off} \geq 8 \times 10^5$. This ratio is easily achieved with the use of a-Si:H TFTs with $I_{on}/I_{off} \sim 10^7$, poly-Si TFTs with $I_{on}/I_{off} \sim 10^6$, or with organic TFTs with $I_{on}/I_{off} \sim 10^8$ (Ref. [70]).

The second requirement is an estimation of the field-effect mobility, μ_{FET}, needed to allow the complete charging of the pixel electrode storage capacitor in the allotted time frame. To make this estimate, the following equation has been developed:

$$\mu_{FET}\frac{W_2}{L_2} \geq \frac{5MC_{pix}}{T_f C_{OX}(V_{GS2} - V_{th})},\tag{5.4}$$

where μ_{FET} is the field effect mobility, W_2 is the width of T_2, L_2 is the length of T2, M is the total number of rows, C_{pix} is the total pixel capacitance, T_f is the frame time, C_{OX} is the insulator layer capacitance, V_{GS2} is the gate to the source voltage of T2, and V_{th} is the threshold voltage of the TFT. A simple calculation with judicious values gives $\mu_{FET} W_2/L_2 \geq 3$ cm^2/V$_s$. Again, this can be accomplished with a-Si:H, poly-Si, and organic TFTs that have reasonable W/L ratios.[70] In order to achieve a pixel brightness of 100 cd/m^2 from a sufficient pixel area, a current of approximately 10^{-7} A is required.

The a-Si:H and poly-Si based TFTs can provide the required ON/OFF current ratio and have carrier mobilities that allow fast switching speeds and charging of the pixel elements. In addition, the TFT needs to have sharp subthreshold slope and must be electrically stable over time. In general, the organic TFTs have insufficient subthreshold slope, and therefore have a high turn-on voltage (tens of volts). Also, they are not very stable electrically. Therefore, the organic TFTs are currently not a practical choice for AMOLEDs. Table 5.4 presents a comparison of typical values of certain parameters for a-Si:H and poly-Si TFTs. It shows that a-Si:H TFTs are capable of supplying the required current, and are therefore capable of driving OLED-based displays. Next, we discuss the technology and fabrication processes used to fabricate a-Si:H and poly-Si TFT AM arrays.

Table 5.4 Comparison of a-Si:H and poly-Si TFT properties.

Property	a-Si:H TFT	poly-Si TFT
Typical mobility (cm^2/V·s)	0.6–1.0	50–100
TFT W/L ratio	10:1	10:1
Maximum current (A)	2.5×10^{-5}	2.1×10^{-3}
Maximum OLED luminance (cd/m^2)	5,000	$>4 \times 10^5$

5.6.1 a-Si:H TFT technology

The fabrication steps of a-Si:H TFTs for a four-TFT AM pixel electrode circuit was described by He et al.[77] The fabrication of this circuit is similar to that of a conventional inverted-staggered, back channel-etched a-Si:H TFT and is shown in Fig. 5.23. The first step is the deposition, by sputtering, of 1000 Å of chromium onto a Corning 1737 glass substrate. This layer is then patterned to form the TFT gate electrodes and the bottom electrode of the storage capacitor (a). Next, a 3000-Å layer of a-SiN$_x$:H, a 2000-Å layer of undoped a-Si:H, and a 500-Å layer of n+ a-Si:H are deposited, respectively, using PECVD (b). The active area of the TFT (a-Si:H) is then defined (c) and gate vias opened (d). Next, a 2000 Å-thick layer of molybdenum is deposited by sputtering and patterned to form the source and drain electrodes of the TFTs and the top electrode of the storage capacitor (e). The TFT is back channel-etched using reactive ion etching (RIE) (e). A 3000 Å-thick layer of a-SiN$_x$:H is deposited as a passivation layer and vias are opened (f). Finally, the electrode material (ITO) is sputtered, annealed, and etched (g).[77] The OLED structure is fabricated on the top of the ITO electrode. In this configuration the light is emitted through glass substrate.

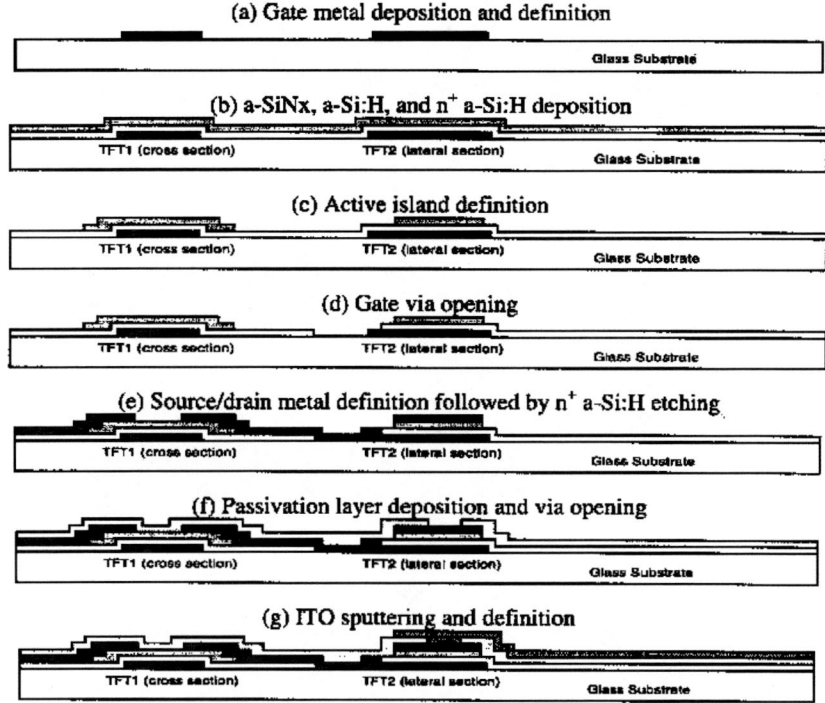

Figure 5.23 Fabrication process for an a-Si:H-based TFT AM pixel.

5.6.2 Poly-Si TFT Technology

Both high-temperature (HT, above 600°C) and low-temperature (LT, below 600°C) poly-Si TFTs are capable of driving high-resolution AMOLEDs. However, only the LT poly-Si TFTs have the capability to be fabricated on large transparent substrates. Therefore, we will describe one of the many LT poly-Si TFT technology and fabrication processes. The cross-sectional structure of the poly-Si TFT AM pixel is shown in Fig. 5.24.[100]

First, a 100-nm amorphous silicon film is deposited using low-pressure chemical vapor deposition (LPCVD). The a-Si:H film is then crystallized by laser annealing. In this approach, the film is irradiated multiple times by a KrF excimer laser to form a poly-crystalline film. The film is then etched to form a poly-Si island. Next, a gate insulator is formed using plasma-enhanced chemical vapor deposition (PECVD) of SiO_2 or a-SiN_x. A poly-Si gate layer is deposited and etched. Next, phosphorous (boron) is implanted to form a self-aligned n-channel (p-channel) TFT. To finish the TFT, a metal (Al) layer is sputtered and etched to form bus lines and a gate, and source and drain connections. The TFT is passivated with an insulating layer, and vias are opened in this layer to allow the contact to the ITO electrode. ITO is deposited and etched to form the anode of the

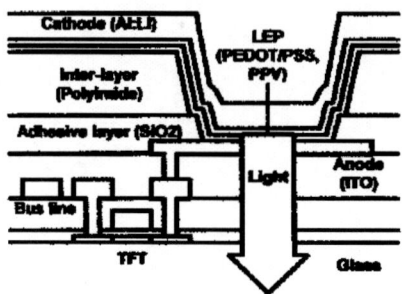

Figure 5.24 Cross section of a poly-Si TFT AM pixel. Reprinted from Ref. [100] with permission of the IEEE.

OLED.[100] Again, the OLED is fabricated over the ITO electrode. In this configuration the light is emitted through glass substrate.

In this pixel circuit, p-channel poly-Si TFTs are used due to good electrical device reliability. In general, it is accepted that the p-channel device is much more electrically stable than the n-channel device.

5.6.3 Pixel electrode circuits

Unlike typical AMLCDs where one TFT is used as a switch, in AMOLEDs at least two TFTs are needed, as shown in Figs. 5.22 and 5.25. One TFT (T1) is used as a switching device and the other TFT (T2) is used as a current-driving device, because a continuous current flow through the pixel_OLED is required during a frame time for a continuous pixel light-emission. As indicated above, the TFTs can be fabricated from a-Si:H or poly-Si thin films. So far, the poly-Si TFT technology has been used most frequently in AMOLEDs because the poly-Si TFTs show better electrical performance (high field-effect mobility) and higher electrical stabil-

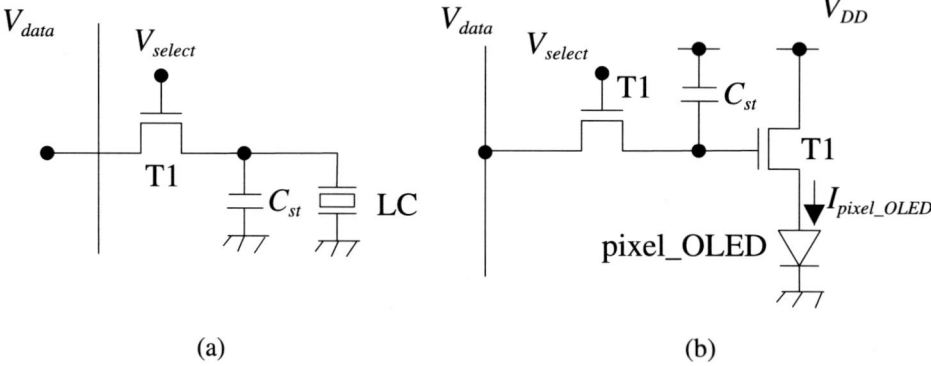

Figure 5.25 An example of the pixel electrode circuit for (a) an AMLCD, and (b) an AMOLED.

Table 5.5 Comparison of LT poly-Si and a-Si:H TFT properties.

Property	LT poly-Si TFT	a-Si:H TFT
Threshold voltage (V)	3–5	~2
Field-effect mobility (cm^2/Vs)	50–120	~1
Off current	$10^{-11} - 10^{-9}$ A	$10^{-13} - 10^{-12}$ A
Maximum process temperature (°C)	550–600	150–300
Driver integration	Yes	Possible
Threshold voltage stability	Good	OK
Mobility and threshold voltage variation over large area	OK	Very good
Manufacturability	Maturing	Very mature
Cost	High	Low
Plastic compatibility	Developing	Good

ity (lower threshold voltage shift) in comparison with a-Si:H TFTs. Table 5.5 shows the electrical performance, advantages, and disadvantages of the LT poly-Si and a-Si:H TFTs for AMOLEDs.[85, 100, 118, 127]

The advantages of LT poly-Si TFTs are as follows:

- A low driving voltage is needed to produce a given current flow through the OLED due to the high TFT field-effect mobility.
- The peripheral driver circuit can be integrated on the display substrates.
- The TFT threshold voltage is stable during display operation.

The disadvantages of LT poly-Si TFTs are as follows:

- The off current is rather high, which can cause an undesirable charge leakage problem through the switching TFT when the pixel is deselected.
- The TFT threshold voltage and field-effect mobility are not uniform over large areas, since laser crystallization is used to produce poly-Si film.
- The manufacturing techniques are expensive and not yet mature.
- The rather high-temperature process may not be compatible with plastic substrates.

The advantages and disadvantages of poly-Si TFTs can, conversely, be the disadvantages and advantages of a-Si:H TFTs. For example, the low driving-current capacity of a-Si:H TFTs, due to their rather low field-effect mobility, has been a significant issue in AMOLEDs that are based on a-Si:H TFT technology. However, dramatic progress made recently in the luminous efficiency of light-emitting organic[72] or polymeric[27, 122] materials has rendered a-Si:H TFT technology as a competing technology in AMOLEDs. Several AMOLED prototypes based on a-Si:H TFT technology have been described recently in the literature.[85, 99, 110]

Although the prototypes of poly-Si and a-Si:H TFT AMOLEDs have already been demonstrated, the device parameter variations of the OLEDs and TFTs are still critical issues for the operation stability of AMOLEDs. The OLED threshold voltage may vary from pixel to pixel after fabrication, then increase slowly at 0.1–1 mV/hour[146] during display operation. The field-effect mobility of both poly-Si and a-Si:H TFTs may vary from pixel to pixel due to either process variations or device aging effects.[85, 146] These effects must be compensated for in an AMOLED in order to obtain a uniform light emission and stable operation of the display. This compensation can be achieved by selecting an appropriate AMOLED pixel electrode circuit configuration based on either voltage-driven[49, 99, 146, 151] or current-driven[50, 56, 84, 132, 147] schemes. In the voltage- and current-driven pixel electrode circuits, voltage and current, respectively, are used as data signals.

Figure 5.25(b) shows a simple voltage-driven pixel electrode circuit with two n-type TFTs. As previously noted, T1 and T2 act as a switching TFT and a driving TFT, respectively. T1 operates in the linear regime and T2 in either the linear or saturation regimes. When V_{select} is high (select time), T1 is on. A data voltage is written onto the storage capacitor (C_{st}) through T1, and the corresponding current (I_{pixel_OLED}) flows from the voltage data-drive, V_{DD}, through T2 to pixel_OLED. Then the pixel will emit light. When V_{select} is low (deselect time), T1 is off and the stored voltage (C_{st}) determines the amount of the current flow through pixel_OLED. Therefore, if there is no change in the stored voltage, the same amount of current flows from V_{DD} through T2 to *pixel_OLED*, producing a continuous pixel light-emission with the same brightness. However, in this simple voltage-driven pixel electrode circuit, I_{pixel_OLED} can vary because the data voltage is a summation of V_{GS_T2} and voltage across the pixel_OLED. This will lead to nonuniform display light-emission if there are any changes in the turn-on voltage of the pixel_OLED and threshold voltage of the TFTs at a given data voltage.[146] Therefore, simple voltage-driven pixel electrode circuits cannot be used in AMOLEDs to produce a uniform brightness level across the whole display.

Based on the simple voltage-driven pixel electrode circuit, researchers at Seiko-Epson Corporation and Cambridge Display Technology[151] reported the area ratio gray scale (ARGS) method to achieve uniform light emission of an AMOLED. They used the poly-Si TFT technology as shown in Fig. 5.26. In the ARGS method, each pixel consists of nine same-dimension subpixels with one n-type (T1) TFT and one p-type (T2) TFT; T1 operates as a switching device and T2 operates as a switch-like driving device. Instead of changing the T2 driving current to produce gray scales as in a simple voltage-driven pixel electrode circuit, in the ARGS method the gray scale is obtained by selecting the number of light-emitting subpixels; thus, 10 gray scales can be achieved with a nine-subpixel structure. The subpixel operates like a binary mode by applying two separate V_{data} values that are either high or low enough to fully turn on and off T2, respectively, no mat-

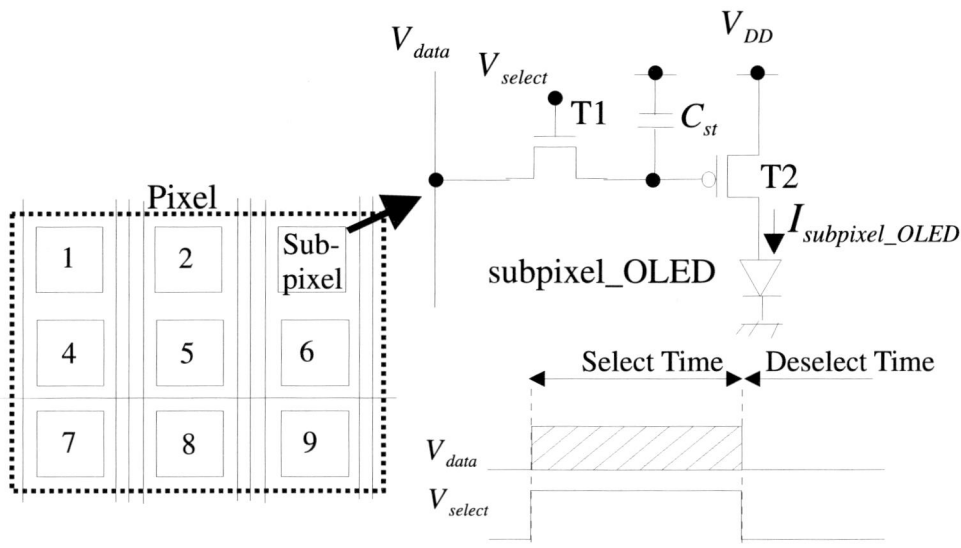

Figure 5.26 Area ratio gray scale (ARGS) method based on a simple voltage-driven AMOLED pixel electrode circuit proposed by Shimoda et al.[150, 151]

ter what change occurs in the T2 threshold voltage. In addition, V_{DD} determines the current level through the subpixel_OLED. Therefore, the T2 threshold voltage shift will not change the current flow through the subpixel_OLED. However, the ARGS method is limited because the number of subpixels determines the possible number of gray scales. To increase the number of gray scales, the ARGS method can be combined with the time ratio gray scale (TRGS) method, which requires a complicated subframe driving scheme and an additional erase scan TFT in each subpixel.[150]

The first voltage-driven pixel electrode circuit with the threshold voltage compensation was reported by Dawson et al.[49] Their circuit consists of four p-type poly-Si TFTs, one selection (V_{select}), and two control lines (AZ and AZB), as shown in Fig. 5.27(a). T1, T3, and T4 are switching TFTs, and T2 is a driving TFT. When V_{select} is low (select time), T1 is on. The select time consists of five subperiods. During periods 1 and 2, $|V_{GS\_T2}|$ is larger than the magnitude of the T2 threshold voltage, $|V_{th\_T2}|$, which is stored across the storage capacitor (C_{st2}). Then, during periods 3 and 4, T2 conducts until $|V_{GS\_T2}|$ is equal to $|V_{th\_T2}|$, storing the V_{th_T2} across C_{st2}. When V_{data} is reduced by ΔV_{data} (period 5), $|V_{GS\_T2}| = |V_{th\_T2}| + |\Delta V_{GS\_T2}|$, $|\Delta V_{GS\_T2}| = (|\Delta V_{data}| \times C_{st1})/(C_{st1} + C_{st2} + C_{G\_T2})$, where C_{G_T2} is the total gate parasitic capacitance of T2. When V_{select} is high (deselect time), T1 is off. The stored V_{GS_T2} is maintained during periods 6 and 7 until T4 is on. Finally, $I_{pixel\_OLED} \propto (\Delta V_{GS\_T2})^2 \propto (\Delta V_{data})^2$ during period 8, which indicates that the current flow through the pixel_OLED depends on ΔV_{data}, not V_{data} or V_{th_T2}. However, this pixel electrode circuit has two control lines, which can make the pixel electrode circuit configuration rather complicated and may cause threshold voltage settling and data voltage writing problems within a row select time.[146]

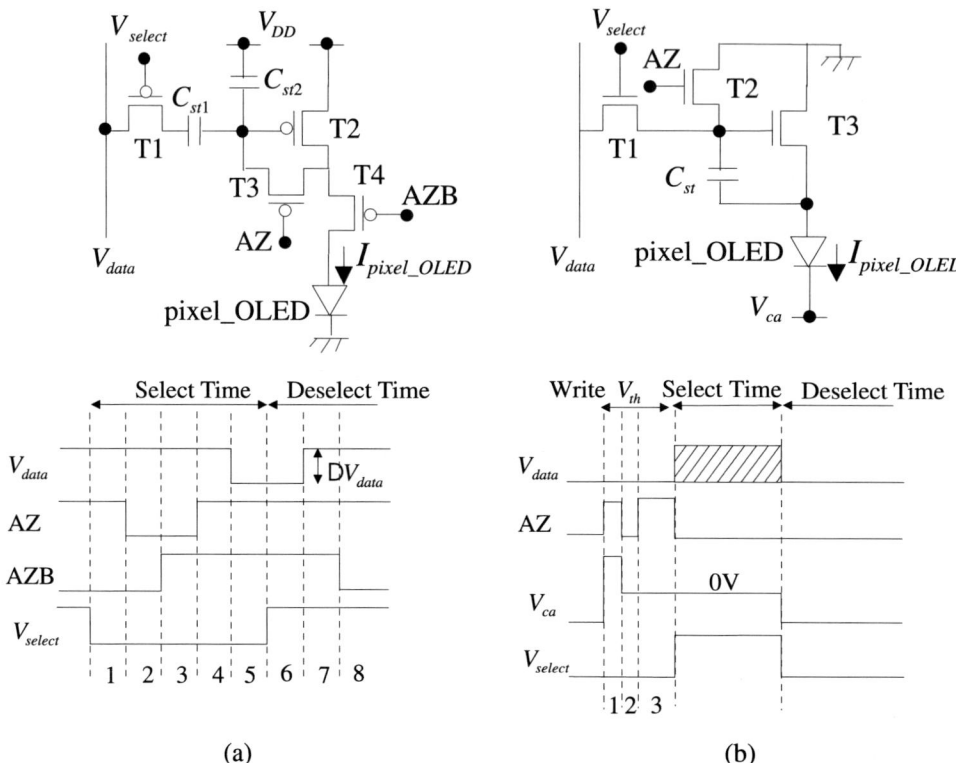

Figure 5.27 Two types of voltage-driven pixel electrode circuits with threshold voltage compensation. The circuit in (a) was proposed by Dawson et al.[49] and the circuit in (b) by Sanford et al.[146]

Another voltage-driven pixel electrode circuit has been reported by Stanford et al.[146] Their circuit consists of three n-type TFTs, one select (V_{select}), one control line (AZ), and one programmable cathode line (V_{ca}), as shown in Fig. 5.27(b). T1 and T2 are switching TFTs, and T3 is a driving TFT. This pixel electrode circuit can compensate for the TFT threshold voltage with the proper signals and timing. Writing the threshold voltage (periods 1 to 3 with V_{select} on low and T1 off) involves three steps. During period 1, while the cathode voltage V_{ca} is negative, the AZ input is high for a short amount of time. This establishes a capacitor voltage that is larger than the T3 threshold voltage. During period 2, V_{ca} is brought to positive voltage and the AZ input is low. T3 conducts, resulting in a negative voltage drop across the pixel_OLED. During period 3, V_{ca} is set at 0 V and the AZ input is set high. T3 conducts until a voltage approximately equal to the T3 threshold voltage is established across the storage capacitor. After this initial threshold voltage establishment, V_{select} is high and T1 is on, and then data voltage is written into the pixel circuit (select time) while V_{ca} is at 0 V and the AZ input is low. The voltage across the storage capacitor will be $V_{data} + V_{th\_T3}$. After data voltage has been written to all the rows in the display, V_{select} is set low and T1 is off (deselect time), and

V_{ca} is brought to a negative voltage. T3 will provide a current flow through the pixel_OLED, which is independent of V_{th_T3} and proportional to $(V_{data})^2$. In this pixel electrode circuit, the pixel_OLED emits the light only after the data voltage writing is finished.

The voltage-driven pixel electrode circuit can successfully compensate for the TFT threshold voltage variation. The operator can also compensate for the pixel_OLED threshold voltage shift by operating the driving TFT in the saturation regime, in which the current flow through the driving TFT (and thus through the pixel_OLED) depends on the V_{GS}, not the V_{DS} (voltage data-source), of the driving TFT. Therefore, although any voltage shift occurs in the pixel_OLED, changing the V_{DS} of the driving TFT will automatically compensate for it, and the current through the pixel_OLED will not change much. However, these voltage-driven driving schemes are limited to TFT threshold voltage compensation and are not adequate to compensate for the TFT field-effect mobility variations.

Several current-driven pixel electrode circuits[50, 56, 84, 132, 147] have been reported to fully compensate for TFT threshold voltage and field-effect mobility variations. In addition, since OLED brightness is directly related to the current flow through the device, the current-driven AM driving method has the benefit of producing a uniform display luminance by delivering current directly onto each pixel.

Dawson et al.[50] reported a current-programmed OLED pixel that consists of four poly-Si p-type TFTs, as shown in Fig. 5.28(a). T1, T3, and T4 are switching TFTs, and T2 is a driving TFT. In this pixel electrode circuit, the data current is written directly onto the pixel, and the corresponding charge will be stored across the storage capacitor. When V_{select} is low and the VGP (the voltage across the fourth transistor) is high (select time), T1 and T3 are on. Then current is provided by I_{data} through T3 and T2 to pixel_OLED, and the pixel_OLED emits light. A specific T2 gate-to-source voltage corresponding to the data current is simultaneously set across the storage capacitor. When V_{select} is high and VGP is low (deselect time), current is provided from V_{DD} through T4 and T2 to pixel_OLED, and pixel_OLED emits light. Since the stored V_{GS_T2} determines the current level during deselect time, the same amount of current flow is guaranteed through the pixel_OLED during the total time frame if T2 operates in the saturation regime.

Toshiba and Matsushita[132] reported a similar current-programmed pixel electrode circuit, as shown in Fig. 5.28(b), which they called a current-copy pixel (CCP). The CCP consists of four p-type poly-Si TFTs. T1, T3, and T4 are switching devices, and T2 is a driving device. When $V_{select1}$ is low and $V_{select2}$ is high (select time), T1 and T3 are on and T4 is off. Current flows from V_{DD} through T2 and T3 to the current source. The storage capacitor is charged during select time. When $V_{select1}$ is high and $V_{select2}$ is low (deselect time), T1 and T3 are off and T4 is on. Current flows from V_{DD} through T2 and T4 to the pixel_OLED. The amount of current during deselect time is determined by the stored voltage across the storage capacitor; thus, the same amount of current flow is again guaranteed if T2 operates in the saturation regime and there is no stored charge variation. The pixel_OLED emits light only during deselect time.

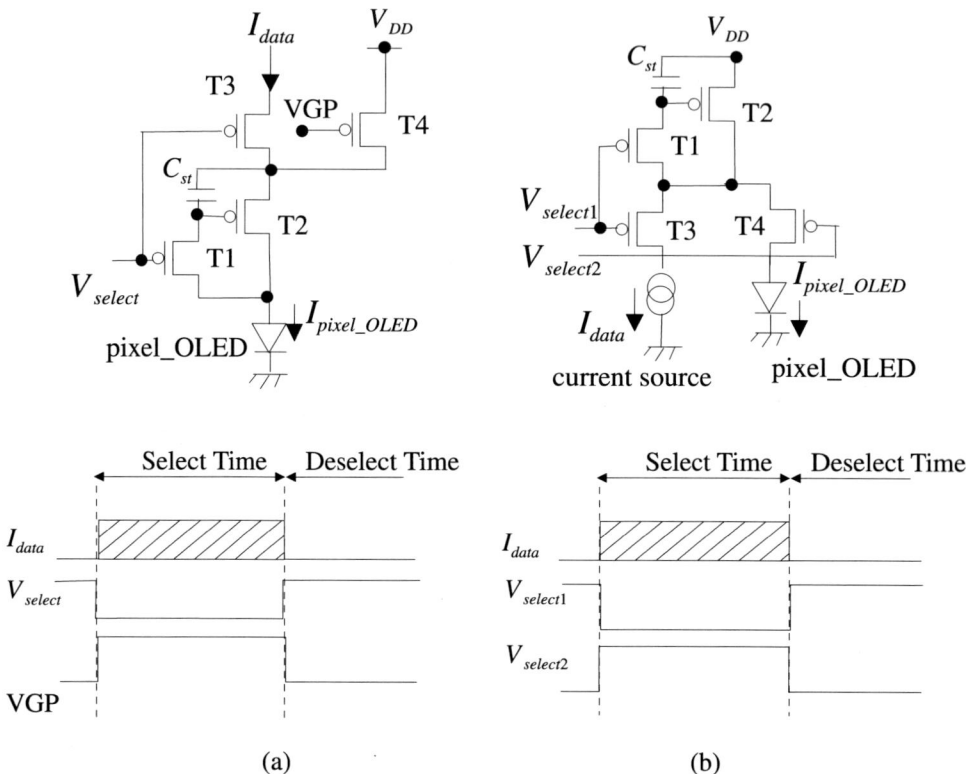

Figure 5.28 Two types of current-programming, current-driven pixel electrode circuits. The circuit in (a) was proposed by Dawson et al.[50] and the circuit in (b) by Ohta et al.[132]

These types of current-programmed OLED pixels may have charging time problems for data current at low gray scales in high-resolution display applications, although they can compensate for both the TFT's threshold voltage and field-effect mobility variations, and for the OLED threshold voltage shift. The data current must first charge up the parasitic capacitance formed between the data lines and cathode before the current is written onto a specific pixel within select time. Therefore, the actual charging process of each pixel cannot be completed within select time since the parasitic capacitance increases as the number of pixels increases.

To solve this charging time issue in current-driven AM driving methods, Sony Corporation[147] introduced a current-mirror type of pixel electrode circuit with two n-type (T3 and T4) and two p-type poly-Si TFTs (T1 and T2), as shown in Fig. 5.29(a). T3 and T4 are switching TFTs, and T1 and T2 form back-to-back transistors of the current mirror. During select time, the write (Write scan) and erase (Erase scan) scan lines are high, and the data current flows from V_{DD} through T1 and T3 to the I_{data} line. At the same time, I_{pixel_OLED} flows from V_{DD} through T2 to pixel_OLED, and the pixel_OLED emits light. By setting the channel width of T1 larger than that of T2, the data current is larger than the I_{pixel_OLED}, which makes the write operation fast enough even at a low gray scale. During deselect time, the write scan is low and

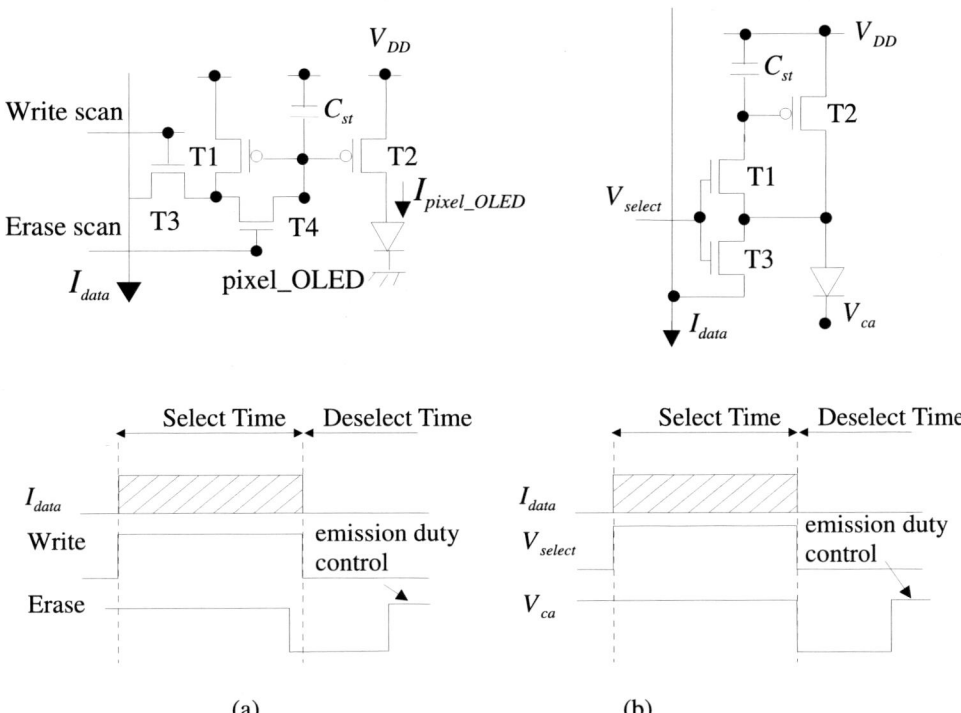

Figure 5.29 Two types of current-mirror, current-driven pixel electrode circuits for AMOLEDs, proposed by (a) Sasaoka et al.[147] and (b) Fish et al.[56]

T1 is off. The same amount of I_{pixel_OLED} continuously flows through the pixel_OLED; a continuous light-emission can be achieved because C_{st} determines the I_{pixel_OLED} level, and T2 operates in the saturation regime during deselect time. Sony introduced an erase scan line to obtain a secure write operation by turning T4 off slightly earlier than T3. The erase scan can also control the time-averaged pixel brightness and the pixel emission duty by turning T4 on during deselect time. The pixel emission duty control produces a high-quality, fast-moving image.

Philips Research Laboratories[56] also reported a modified current-mirror type of pixel electrode circuit with two n-type and one p-type poly-Si TFTs, as shown in Fig. 5.29(b). T1 and T3 are switching TFTs, and T2 is a driving TFT. During select time, V_{select} is high, T1 and T3 are on, and the data current flows from V_{DD} through T1 and T3 to the I_{data} line, thus charging C_{st} to a level corresponding to the data-current level. No current flows through pixel_OLED because V_{ca} is high during select time. Then, during deselect time, V_{select} is low, T1 and T3 are off, the same amount of current flows from V_{DD} through T2 to the pixel_OLED, and pixel_OLED emits light. The stored charge in the storage capacitor determines the current level, and T2 operates in the saturation regime during deselect time. Philips used a pulsed cathode voltage approach (V_{ca}) to operate the pixel electrode circuit at an efficient pixel_OLED operating point. This pulsed cathode voltage approach has other advantages, such

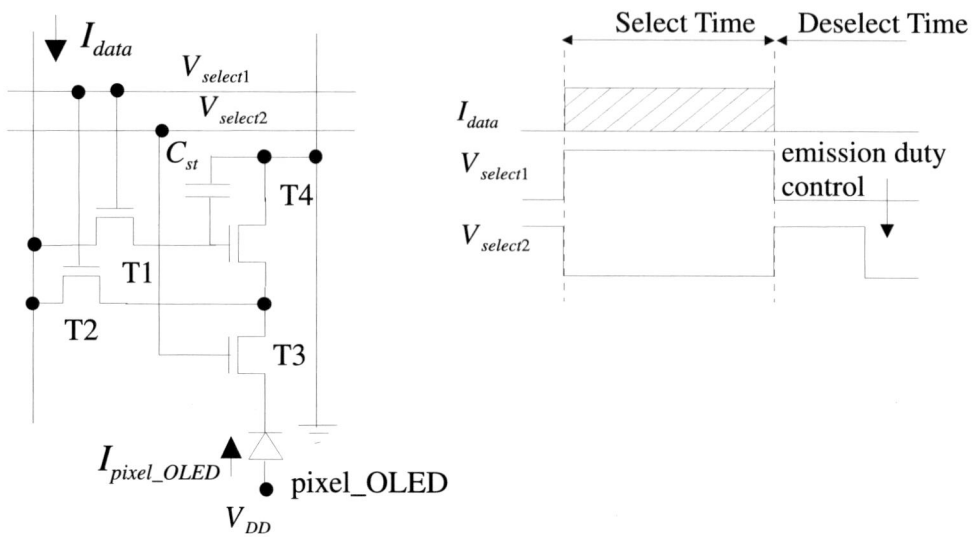

Figure 5.30 A current-sink, current-driven pixel electrode circuit proposed by Hong et al.[83]

as a higher programming current and an emission duty control for an improved motion image.

Kanicki's research group[83] also reported a current-sink pixel electrode circuit with four n-type poly-Si TFTs, as shown in Fig. 5.30. T1 and T2 are selecting TFTs, and T3 and T4 are switching and driving TFTs, respectively. The T1/T2 and T3 TFTs control the current flow path according to appropriate selecting voltage signals. During select time, T1and T2 are on and T4 is off, directing the data current flow from the data line to the source line (GND) through T2 and T3. After the storage capacitor is charged up during select time, the $V_{select1}$ and $V_{select2}$ signals change during frame time, turning T1 and T2 off and T4 on, respectively. Then the data current will flow from V_{DD} to ground through the OLED, T_3, and T_4. The $V_{select2}$ waveform can be appropriately selected for a higher programming current and an emission duty control, which produces a high-quality, fast-moving image. This pixel electrode circuit requires a top-anode pixel_OLED structure as shown in Fig. 5.31(b).

It is noted that all the above voltage-driven and current-driven pixel electrode circuits are based on poly-Si TFT technology. For large-area, low-cost, high-resolution displays, the poly-Si TFT AMOLED can be challenged by a low-cost a-Si:H TFT AMOLED based on the AM arrays developed for AMLCDs. One example of such a pixel electrode circuit is shown in Fig. 5.32. This a-Si:H TFT circuit was developed in Kanicki's research group.[85] The four-TFT pixel circuit can provide continuous current even after the pixel is deselected; and the TFT threshold voltage variations, which occur due to process variations and operational stress, are fully compensated in this circuit. The circuit has four external connections: V_{DD}, V_{select}, I_{data}, and ground (also the OLED cathode). As shown in the figure, TFT T5 and C_{diode} are used to schematically represent the OLED.

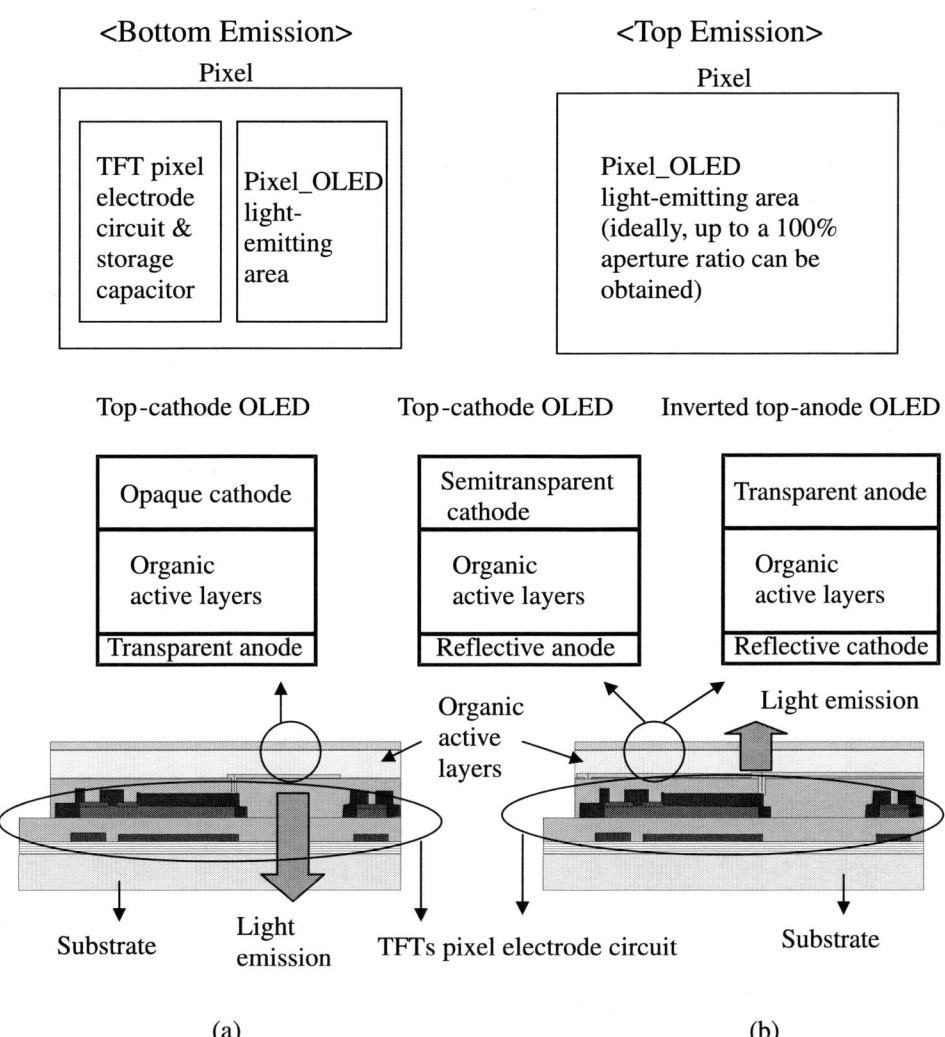

Figure 5.31 Bottom-emission and top-emission pixel electrode circuit configurations.

First we will describe the "on" (pixel selected) state. When the V_{select} signal is made high, the switching TFTs, T1 and T2, are turned on. The data signal current, from I_{data}, passes through T1 and T2, thereby storing charge on the storage capacitor and setting the drain and gate biases of the drive TFT (T3). This allows the data current to pass through T3. The value of V_{DD} has been chosen so that it is lower than the bias on the drain of T3, ensuring that no current can flow through TFT T4. This guarantees that all of the data current, I_{data}, which passes through T3, then goes through T5 (OLED) to ground. When the pixel is deselected (the "on" state), the select line bias is made low. This turns the switching TFTs, T1 and T2, off. The charge on the storage capacitor maintains the bias on the gate of T3. Therefore, current still flows through T3, causing the bias on the drain of T3 to

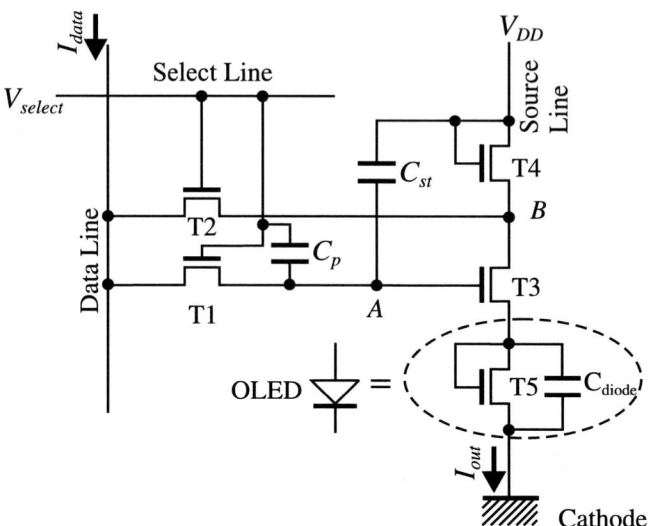

Figure 5.32 Equivalent pixel electrode circuit of a four a-Si:H TFT proposed by He et al.[75, 77] © J. Kanicki.

drop rapidly. When the bias on the drain of T3 drops below V_{DD}, T4 will turn on and maintain a constant current through T3. In this state, the current flows from V_{DD}, through T4 and T3, and then through T5 (OLED) to ground. Even in the "on" state, the required data current through the OLED is maintained. [76, 84]

It is possible, through process variations and operational device stress, that the threshold voltage of the drive transistor T3 can change. The four-TFT pixel circuit can compensate for such changes through the following mechanisms. Since T1, T2, and T4 are used as switches and are not used to control the output current, threshold voltage variations in these TFTs will not affect the output current.[77] However, if the threshold voltage of T3 changes, the gate bias must be changed in order to maintain the desired amount of output current. Since I_{data} is forced through T3, the gate voltage of T3 adjusts to maintain this amount of current, regardless of the value of the threshold voltage. Therefore, the threshold voltage variation of T3 will not affect the level of output current.[77, 78] This pixel electrode circuit with some modifications, as described in Ref. [78], was used to produce a-Si:H TFT current-driven AMOLEDs.[85, 86] This driving pixel electrode circuit showed the ability to provide a pixel electrode brightness in excess of 1000 cd/m^2 for a typical OLED with an external efficiency of 1%.

Although each pixel electrode circuit has its advantages and disadvantages, their operating principles can be categorized under two main types—voltage-driven and current-driven AMOLED driving schemes—as shown in Table 5.6. In both driving schemes, the driving TFT typically operates in the saturation regime to compensate for voltage variations. The voltage-driven pixel electrode circuits can be combined easily with a commercially available AMLCD data voltage driver. However, as previously noted, they are limited to fully compensating for TFT

Table 5.6 Comparison between voltage-driven and current-driven AMOLED driving schemes.

Property	Voltage-driven AMOLED	Current-driven AMOLED
Data signal	Voltage	Current
Data signal driver	Commercially available (AMLCD driver can be used)	Under development (standardization may be required)
Slow charging time an issue at low display brightness levels?	No	Yes (can be solved by current-mirror or current-sink type structure)
TFT threshold voltage compensation?	Yes (complicated threshold voltage memory steps are required during select time)	Yes
TFT field-effect mobility compensation?	No	Yes
OLED threshold voltage compensation?	Yes (by the driving TFT)	Yes (by both the driving TFT and direct current writing)

field-effect mobility variations. In addition, rather complicated control signals are required to write the TFT threshold voltage information onto each pixel. For the current-driven pixel electrode circuits, specific data current drivers are needed for each pixel electrode circuit configuration. The magnitude of data current depends upon the display format and pixel electrode circuit design. Therefore, standardizing data current drivers is required for the commercial applications of the current-driven pixel electrode circuits, which may be very challenging. The issue of a slow charge at a low display brightness in the current-driven pixel electrode circuit can be solved by introducing a current-mirror and/or a current-sink type of pixel electrode structure. However, the direct writing of data current onto each pixel is a big advantage of the current-driven pixel electrode circuits, which can fully compensate for not only TFT and OLED threshold voltage shifts, but also for TFT field-effect mobility variations.

The pixel configuration is determined by the OLED structure. A typical OLED structure consists of a transparent anode, active organic layers, and an opaque cathode, which is necessary due to the process compatibility of the organic layers and the low work function of the metal cathode. Therefore, most of the mentioned pixel electrode circuits are combined with the opaque top-cathode structure; thus, the light emission is observed through the bottom transparent anode, as shown in Fig. 5.31(a). The bottom-emission type of pixel configuration has a limited pixel aperture ratio, which is closely related to the display power consumption and stability. The aperture ratio is defined by the ratio of the light-emitting area to the total pixel area. To increase the aperture ratio, Sony Corporation[147] adopted a top-emission type of pixel configuration by using an opaque bottom-anode and semitransparent top-cathode pixel structure, as shown in Fig. 5.31(b). Ideally, this approach can produce up to a 100% aperture ratio. Since the light emission in this approach is observed through the semitransparent cathode, a certain amount of light will be lost. Therefore, if an equivalent OLED performance is obtained for an inverted device structure (opaque cathode/active organic layers/transparent anode) in comparison with the conventional OLED structure, the top-emission pixel configuration with a transparent top-anode pixel_OLED structure could be very beneficial for future AMOLEDs. The current-sink type of pixel electrode circuit[83] can also be combined with this transparent top-anode structure, as shown in Fig. 5.31(b).

5.7 Methods to Improve AMOLED Contrast Ratio

The high reflectance of the OLED metal alloy cathode can lead to a low pixel contrast ratio (PCR) in high-ambient illuminance.[70] Here, we quantify the PCR by defining the discrimination ratio as the ratio of the brightness of an "on" pixel to that of an "off" pixel. The brightness of an "off" OLED is taken to be solely due to the reflection of the ambient illuminance, E_a, which is assumed to have a uniform angular distribution. Therefore, the "off" pixel brightness is $L_{off} = RE_a/2\pi$, where R is the reflectance of the pixel measured from the substrate side. The "on" pixel brightness is $L_{on} = L_d + L_{off}$. The discrimination ratio is, therefore, $D = 1 + (2\pi L_d/ RE_a)$, which is plotted in Fig. 5.33 as a function of display reflectance R under $E_a = 500$ lux (ANSI standard) for different display brightnesses (L_d). For $L_d = 100$ cd/m^2 and $R = 80\%$, $D = 2.6$. Discrimination ratios larger than 5 can only be achieved with a display brightness larger than 200 cd/m^2 for high-reflectance pixels under specific ambient lighting conditions. To increase D, the reflection of ambient light must be suppressed.

A circular polarizer (CP) can be placed in front of the display to achieve high discrimination ratios. Although the quarter-wave plate in the CP is wavelength dependent, the reflected ambient light can be sufficiently attenuated if the quarter-wave plate is centered near $\lambda = 555$ nm, where $V(\lambda)$ (the relative spectral luminous efficiency function for photopic vision) is maximum. This is due to the broad spectral width of the CP blocking band coupled with the eye's insensitivity to the wavelengths in the tails of $V(\lambda)$. A 0th-order quarter-wave plate is desirable to obtain a broad blocking band for the CP.

To analyze the improvement in PCR associated with proposed schemes, it is assumed that the front surface of the display is AR coated, and thus the Fresnel reflections at this surface can be neglected. Here, the front of the display is the polarizer surface facing the viewer. Assuming a uniform spectral distribution for the ambient illuminance, a zeroth-order quarter-wave plate centered at $\lambda = 555$ nm and a 100% efficiency for the CP, the luminance due to reflected ambient light is found to be attenuated by a factor of 71, while the emitted light is attenuated by

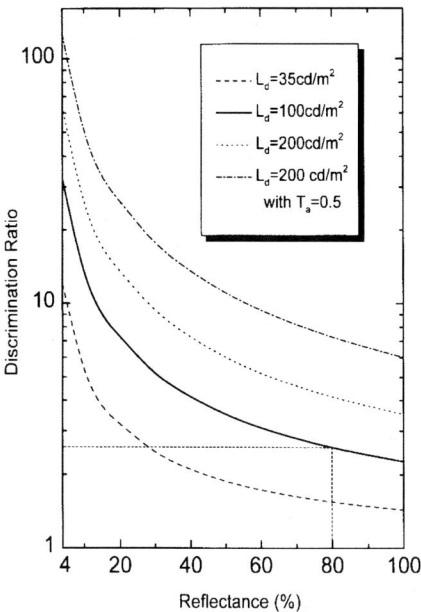

Figure 5.33 Discrimination ratio versus OLED reflectance curves under a 500-lux ambient illuminance. Reprinted from Ref. [70] with permission of the IEEE.

only a factor of 2. Hence, for a display with $L_d = 200$ cd/m^2 (corresponding to a 100 cd/m^2 perceived brightness) and 80% efficiency under a 500-lux ambient illuminance, D is increased to 113.

5.8 Current Market and Future Trends

According to one source,[40] FPDs are a potential $20 billion (U.S. currency) annual market, with about 50% in wireless applications. FPD applications include cell phones, personal digital assistants (PDAs), monitors, and televisions. Annual growth is projected to be 15 to 30% depending on the specific application. In five years, experts estimate that the market could reach $55 billion. According to a display market research firm, Stanford Resources, the worldwide OLED display market is forecasted to increase from several hundred thousand units valued at $3 million in 1999 to more than 100 million units valued at $714 million in 2005. Table 5.7 shows the current and future OLED markets by application.

5.8.1 Comparison between OLED and non-LED displays

The light output of an OLED display is Lambertian, which means the user can view the display from any angle (up to 160 deg) with the same perceived brightness. LCDs, however, are non-Lambertian displays whose image interference pat-

Table 5.7 Worldwide OLED market[a] by application.[b]

Application	2000	2001	2002	2003	2004	2005
Audio	1161	2712	4174	6078	8109	8822
Automobile displays	373	1587	3158	6028	10,035	12,868
Cell phones	60	277	1058	2387	3998	5678
Appliances	1037	2870	6909	13,484	20,656	26,091
Meters/multimeters	910	2005	3495	4776	5745	7220
ATM/cash registers	520	2102	4923	8401	11,474	15,958
Telephones	130	889	1630	2911	4251	6713
Test equipment	360	576	975	1477	2089	2428
VCR/cable boxes	229	1053	2257	3600	5298	7251

[a] Unit shipments given in thousands.

[b] Adapted from Ref. [119] with permission of iSuppli/Stanford Resources.

tern changes as the viewer's eye moves. The eye then perceives a different image, including a different color balance.

OLED displays are low-power displays that use thin organic films as the light emitters, thereby eliminating the need for power-hungry backlights and their environmentally unfriendly mercury content. In conventional LCDs, the backlights are on all the time at full power; but with OLEDs, the individual pixels are turned on and off as they are needed, thereby using only approximately half the power consumption of an LCD. In addition, LCDs are not photoactive. They act as light filters and require back lighting. Only 30 to 35% of the backlight passes through an LCD. As a result, LCDs consume a tremendous amount of power: up to 60% of the drain on a laptop battery is from the LCD.

Currently, efficiencies of the best doped-polymer and molecular OLEDs already exceed that of incandescent light bulbs. Efficiencies of 20 lm/W have been reported for yellow- and green-emitting polymer devices, and 40 lm/W has been attained for phosphorescent molecular OLEDs—compared to less than 20 lm/W for a typical incandescent light bulb. It is reasonable to predict that soon, efficiencies of 80 lm/W (a value comparable to that of fluorescent room lighting) will be achieved using phosphorescent OLEDs.

Not only does the lack of a backlight in OLEDs lengthen the battery life and minimize heat and electric interference, but it also reduces the overall size and weight of the end product. As glass-based displays, LCDs are prone to breakage and can be heavy for small portable applications. A complete poly-OLED display is less than 2 mm thick, weighs approximately 0.1 ounces, and requires a low operating voltage of only 2 to 6 V.

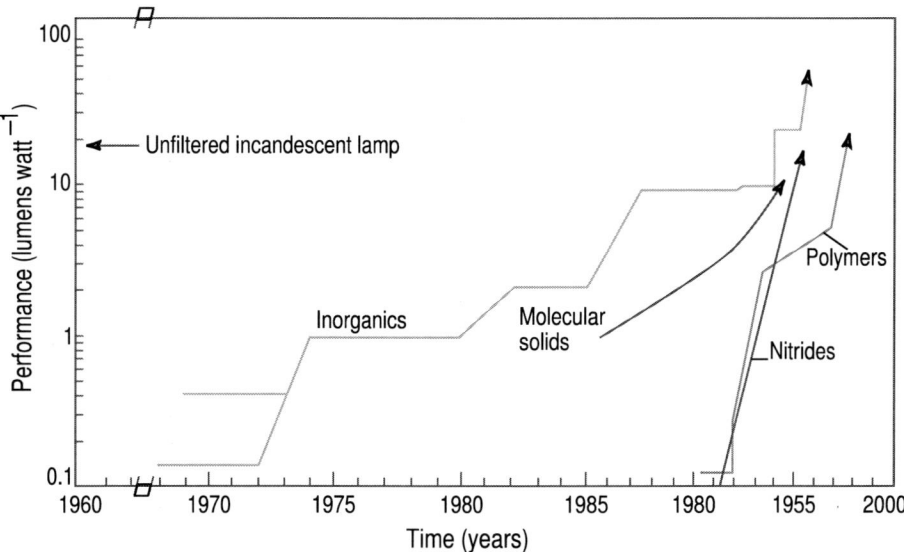

Figure 5.34 Comparison between OLEDs and inorganic LEDs. Reprinted from Ref. [171] with permission of Nature/Macmillan.

5.8.2 Comparison between OLEDs and inorganic LEDs

LEDs based on crystalline inorganic semiconductors have a long history, and their performance has improved steadily since their invention. It is when viewed in this context that the recent progress made with semiconducting organic materials seems so remarkable.

Figure 5.34 shows the evolution of organic and inorganic LEDs with performance given in lumens per watt (a typical value for an unfiltered incandescent lamp is shown for comparison). Inorganic LEDs based on III-V semiconductors such as gallium arsenide arrived on the scene in the early 1960s, and their performance has shown steady but significant progress since that time. Organic LEDs appeared much more recently, yet are already approaching the best performance levels of their inorganic counterparts. The nitride-based semiconductors are another success story and have extended applications of inorganic LEDs into the blue-violet region of the spectrum.

5.8.3 Current and future challenges

Even though OLED display technology enjoys tremendous advantages over traditional inorganic LED and other display technologies such as LCDs, it is not yet ready for batch fabrication and a competitive display market. Several challenges must be overcome.

First, manufacturing difficulties must be reduced.[64] Researchers have encountered many difficulties in manufacturing devices with the thin layers needed to achieve operating voltages between 5 and 10 V. OLEDs are vulnerable to electrical shorts caused by pinhole defects in the film or contamination of the substrate surface by dust particles. Furthermore, the materials tend to be mechanically fragile and are easily attacked by the chemicals used in photolithographic patterning. Therefore, patterning often requires low-resolution methods such as defining the device contact by metal deposition through a shadow mask, often in combination with costly dry-processing techniques. In the future, however, many new lithographic patterning techniques could appear, and even techniques borrowed from other industries such as injection molding, direct imprinting using stamping, and ink-jet printing.

Second, researchers are racing to find ways to effectively combine OLEDs that emit at different color bands into a single full-color display. This is a formidable task. The materials are generally better suited for the deposition of large-area, uniform layers rather than intricately patterned arrays of differently colored pixels; and the emission colors (and efficiencies) of the individual pixels need to be carefully balanced to match the spectral response of the eye. For the molecular systems, vacuum deposition through a patterned "mask" provides a promising route for achieving the necessary control. Prototype 5- to 20-in. displays based on this approach were exhibited by many different companies. Solution-based polymers are not amenable to vapor-phase deposition, so alternative strategies must be explored. The ink-jet technique (as used in color printers) is one possible avenue for producing the necessary pixel arrays, although the initial results suggest that further optimization of this process is needed.

Third, the display market is already well served by several more established technologies, so competition will be stiff. For the cruder monochrome applications, the combination of low power consumption, simplicity of fabrication, and the "gimmick" factor of having an unusually colored display could well be sufficient to give organic LEDs a competitive edge. The situation with full-color displays is harder to predict and, in the short term, they will need to demonstrate a cost advantage if they are to succeed. But in the long term, properties unique to the organic systems (as discussed in previous sections) may come to the fore, and as mentioned above, it is conceivable that within five years, we will have flexible color displays that can be rolled up and put in our pockets.

Finally, although current efforts for commercialization of OLED technology are focused on flat-panel displays, other applications are being investigated. The OLED technology could be used for outdoor and emergency lighting conditions and should be capable of running on full speed at very low temperatures (–40°C or less). This display technology could also be used for cell phones, digital still cameras, camcorders, personal digital assistants, head-wearable displays, and car navigation systems. Also, today flexible OLEDs are being heavily investigated so that one day e-books based on AMOLED technology can substitute for the paper-version books that have been used for thousands of years.

Chapter 6
Display Image Quality Metrics

Good display metrology is reproducible, robust, unambiguous, extensible, distinct, accommodating, accessible, simple, meaningful, and honest.

—Edward F. Kelley

The assessment of display image quality requires the measurement of a number of characteristics that contribute to the fidelity of the image presentation. A complete description of all possible display measurement methods would be extensive and is out of the scope of this tutorial book. Our goal is to focus on the description of the methodology to assess those aspects of display performance that are relevant to medical imaging applications as they affect the medical decision outcome. In this chapter, we discuss the following topics: luminance response at normal and off-normal viewing angles, small-spot contrast ratio, spatial resolution, noise, and reflectance. Other aspects of display performance that are relevant to image quality and must be considered include geometrical distortions, color rendition, and temporal response. For a discussion on measurement methods for some of the latter, readers are referred to Refs. [58] and [143]. Our discussion of the methods for display characterization will include advanced techniques as well as practical aspects.

6.1 Luminance Response

As a general rule, the display brightness should be set to the maximum possible to avoid the natural reduced contrast performance experienced by the human eye in dark regions. The ratio of the maximum-to-minimum luminance should be about 250 to match the range of equalized visual response (see Chapter 2). The maximum luminance (L_{max}) is typically set to a manufacturer-recommended value based on maximizing brightness while controlling spot size and aging. The minimum luminance (L_{min}) should be about four times the luminance resulting from ambient illuminance to provide enough contrast modulation at the lowest luminance values. For consistent gray-scale presentation, the luminance as a function of gray level should follow recommended profiles (i.e., DICOM Part 3.14; see Ref. [2]).

Before performing measurements of the display, the contrast and brightness controls should be set to a particular optimal value, if possible. On many systems, these are accessed only by service tools. Some systems may have an internal photometer to set the brightness and contrast. Some displays may have an illuminance meter in one of the CRT bulb walls, beyond the emissive structure, with which measurements of ambient illumination can be made automatically. The same sensor can be placed beyond the LC cell in AMLCD displays. This is a useful tool, especially if room illumination conditions vary. Otherwise, this measurement can be performed once at the acceptance testing stage or initial display calibration.

The brightness of available display devices varies greatly (see Table 6.1). Monochrome medical devices are substantially brighter than desktop computer displays. With the display's power turned off, the surface of a display device will have a luminance proportional to the ambient illumination level (L_{amb}). This is described by the diffuse reflection coefficient, R_D, in cd/m^2/lux (see Table 6.2)[*]. We established in Chapter 2 that for good performance, L_{amb} should be less than 20% of L_{min}. If $R_D = 0.02$ cd/m^2/lux and $L_{min} = 2.0$ cd/m^2, the ambient illumination should be no greater than 20 lux ($L_{amb} = 20 \times 0.02 = 0.4$ cd/m^2). This is typical of a moderately lit room such as a diagnostic reading area.

Table 6.1 Maximum and minimum luminance of typical display devices.

Display Type	L_{max} (cd/m^2)	L_{min} (cd/m^2)
Generic desktop	85	0.3
Clinical radiologic	250	1.0
Diagnostic radiologic	500	2.0
Transilluminated film	2000	8.0

Table 6.2 Diffuse reflection coefficients for typical display devices.

Display Type	R_D (cd/m^2/lux)
Generic desktop	0.03
Medical monochrome	0.02
Conventional monochrome	0.06
LCD desktop	0.02
Avionics LCD	0.005

---

[*] The definition for the reflection coefficients is introduced in Sec. 6.5.

Display devices require luminance calibration, which involves hardware and software operations. The calibration procedure is aimed at defining what types of luminance transfer characteristics are used for the presentation of gray-scale images. The luminance response can be modified by a software lookup table that converts the display values to modified color map entries. Some display controllers use a photometer to measure luminance and to deduce lookup calibration tables that can be stored in the controller. Software calibration is limited by the number of gray-scale bits available in the visual class and by the controller DAC. Hardware calibration can be achieved by the incorporation of a correction table loaded into the display controller. Display controllers are available that map 8-bit gray values to 10-bit values, or 10-bit values to 12-bit values.

6.1.1 Luminance calibration

The luminance response is defined as the relationship between the image value introduced to the controller and the actual screen luminance. The basic luminance response curve should be measured using a test pattern having a central target and a uniform field (e.g., TG18-LN[143]—see Fig. 6.1). It should be measured with a photometer under conditions of minimal ambient illumination, and the ambient illumination should be separately measured with typical ambient conditions. The results can then be adjusted for the measured contribution of ambient illumination by adding a constant compensation factor to the entire table such that L_{min} is above L_{amb}. As discussed in the previous paragraphs, this factor should satisfy the condition that L_{min} should be equal to or greater than five times the luminance generated by diffuse reflections of ambient illumination. The measured results should be compared to the expected response (e.g., DICOM Part 3.14 standard) with the JND units scaled to match the display values for L_{max} and L_{min}.

It is useful to convert those results to contrast so they can be compared with the expected contrast response (see Figs. 6.1 and 6.2). The contrast metric $(\Delta L/L)^i_{per\ JND}$ is computed for both the expected and the measured responses as the ratio of $\Delta L/L$ divided by the number of JND index values associated with the two luminance values contributing to ΔL.[12]

A standard pattern for measuring the luminance response is needed because the measured luminance response can be contaminated with light coming out of the field of view of the photometer. To illustrate this point, Fig. 6.3 presents the measurement results of L_{min} for a typical monochrome CRT with targets of different sizes. Even though we used a specially collimated probe,[8] L_{min} varies greatly with target size due to the display's veiling glare.

There is no agreement as to what level of deviation from the expected response is acceptable in displays used for diagnosis. As a first approximation, we claim that acceptable levels are less than a 10% deviation for primary displays and less than a 20% deviation for secondary displays. These figures must be associated with a L_{max} of more than 170 cd/m^2 for primary displays, and more than 100 cd/m^2 for secondary

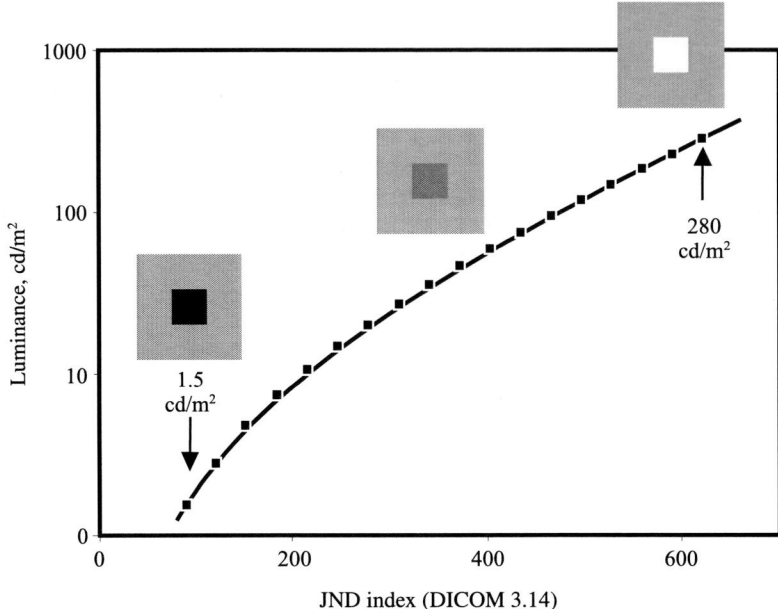

Figure 6.1 Gray-scale display function according to the DICOM Part 3.14 standard function resulting in an increased contrast at low luminance. The inserts show the image patterns used for the measurement of the luminance response with constant background intensity and a centered target.

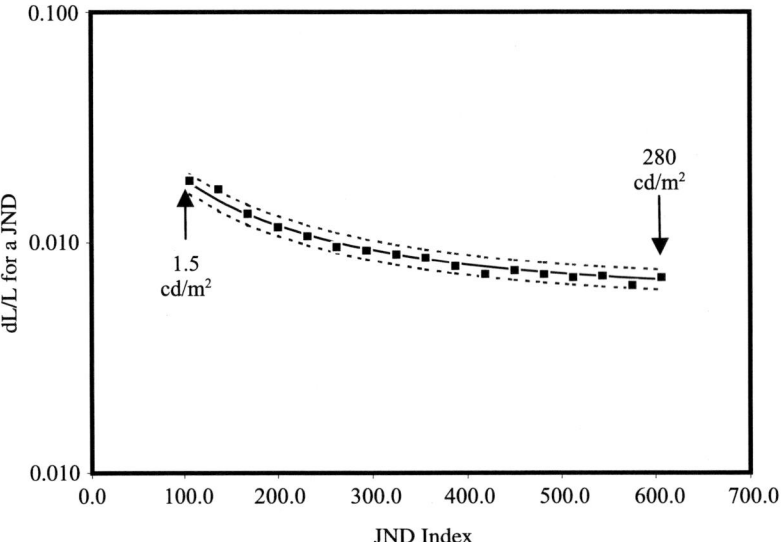

Figure 6.2 Same data presented in Fig. 6.1 but expressed in terms of the change in contrast at each JND level. The solid line represents the expected response according to the calibration performed on this display, and the dotted lines represent the 10% tolerance limits.

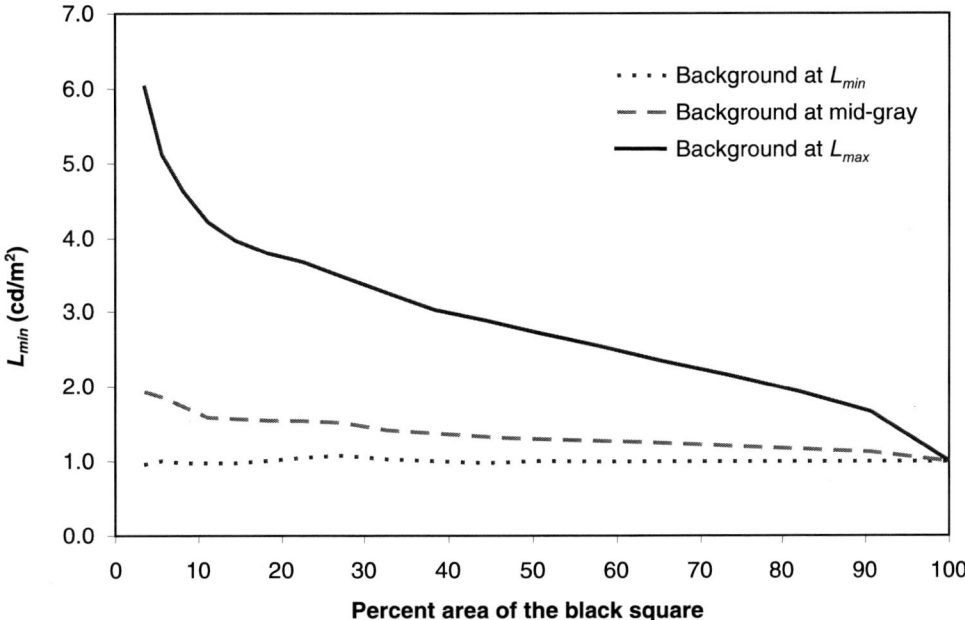

Figure 6.3 Variation of L_{min} measurements for a display having veiling glare. Although the target is at all times driven at the setting for L_{min}, the actual measured luminance changes as the background gray level changes from 1 to 127, and to 255.

displays. The tolerance range for these values can be on the order of 5%. For the L_{min}, an appropriate setting is four times the luminance generated by diffuse ambient reflections to within 10% of the desired value. The luminance range L_{max}/L_{min} should be more than 250 for primary displays, and more than 100 for secondary displays.

A complete description of the luminance response can be made by measuring the luminance output for all digital display values. This is greatly facilitated by the use of a photometer connected to the display workstation and software for automated data acquisition, as schematized in Fig. 6.4. Evaluation of the difference in log-luminance between each digital value can reveal artifacts in contrast transfer. For instance, it is possible that with poor calibration, some unity steps in the digital value scale can yield no change in the luminance output. An example of the evaluation of all 256 levels is presented in Fig. 6.5, which shows that for a calibrated CRT, a unit gray-level increment may cause large changes in the luminance output while other unit gray-level increments bring about only small changes in the luminance.

6.1.2 Angular emission

The angular emission of CRTs is known to be quasi-Lambertian.[5] However, as described in Chapter 4, luminous emissions from AMLCDs are far from being Lambertian. Moreover, they differ from one AMLCD design to the other. A change

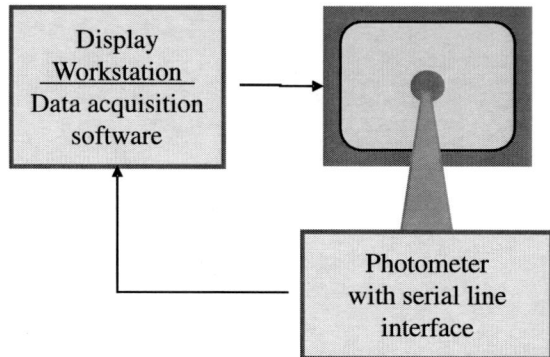

Figure 6.4 Setup for automatic measurement of luminance response.

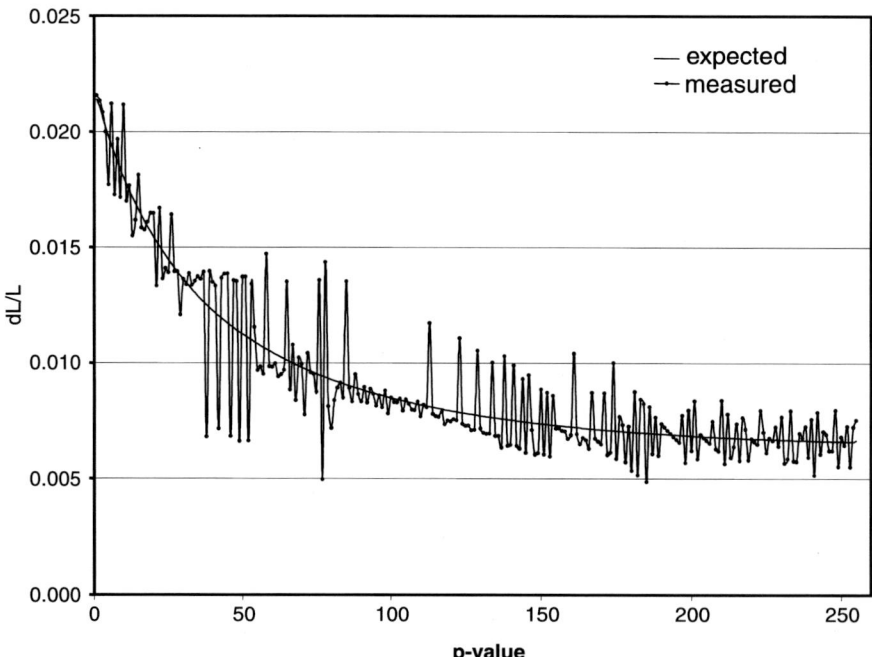

Figure 6.5 Complete evaluation of the luminance response across the 256 gray levels (p-values).

in the angular luminance profile implies that the luminance calibration that was performed on-axis is no longer valid at off-axis angles. It is for this reason that the measurement of angular luminance is relevant to the medical imaging community and is included in this book.

Two distinct methods can be used to measure the angular luminance profiles of a display device.[12] The first method relies on small-spot luminance measurements using a conic collimated photopic probe positioned with a manual rotation arm (see Fig. 6.6). The conic probe measures luminance with a small field of view

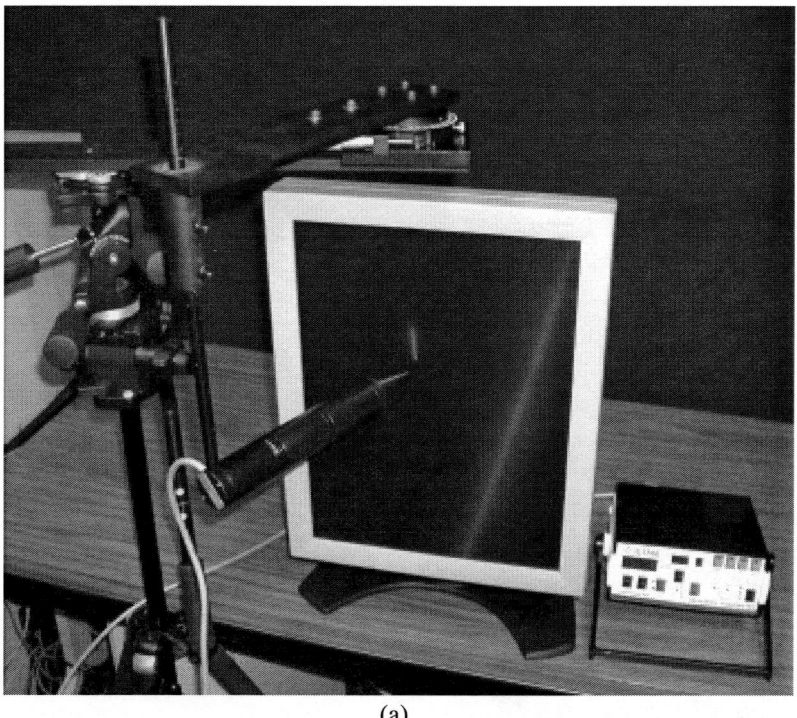

(a)

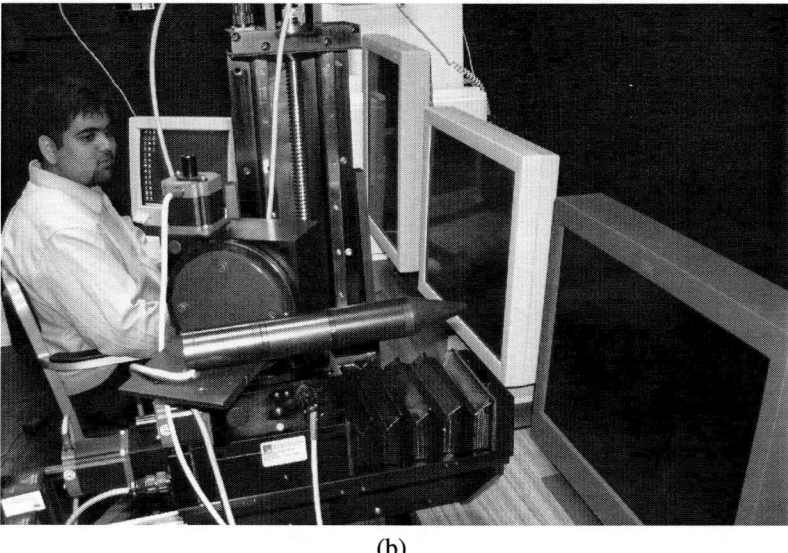

(b)

Figure 6.6 Experimental setup to measure luminance as a function of the viewing direction. The rotation arm shown in (a) allows the user to measure luminance coming from a small spot in the display along an arc, maintaining the same distance between the probe and the spot at all angles. The same measurements can be performed automatically with a five-axis stage controlled via a computer program [shown in (b)] that will display the patterns on the monitor, position the probe at the desired angle, and record the luminance.

and provides optical shielding from emissions at other viewing directions that contaminate the readings.[8] This is especially critical at large, off-normal angles where the luminance measurement would be corrupted by light coming from regions of the display that are closer to the probe (far away from the desired measurement spot), representing a completely different viewing direction with respect to the one we intend to measure.

The probe is connected to a research radiometer with automatic readout. It can be controlled with a software application that displays the 256 gray levels in a square target (10% of the field) with a constant background (at 20% of L_{max}), and acquires 18 consecutive luminance readings. The data containing the average and the standard deviation of the 18 measurements are transferred to a computer file. The results can be analyzed with respect to their departure from the DICOM Part 3.14 gray-scale display function (GSDF)[2] by computing the normalized contrast ($\Delta L/L$) as a function of the JND index, and plotting the experimental data points along with the expected response and the 10% and 25% tolerance limits (see Fig. 6.7). The expected response is calculated by assigning a luminance value for each JND level that is obtained using the DICOM Standard Display Function found on page 16, Annex B of Ref. [2]. The contrast metric $(\Delta L/L)^i_{per\ JND}$ associated with the expected and the measured responses is computed by calculating the ratio of the relative change in luminance over the luminance at each interval, and dividing that number by the number of JNDs in that interval:

$$(\Delta L/L)^i_{per\ JND} = \frac{L_{i+1} - L_i}{JND_{i+1} - JND_i}. \tag{6.1}$$

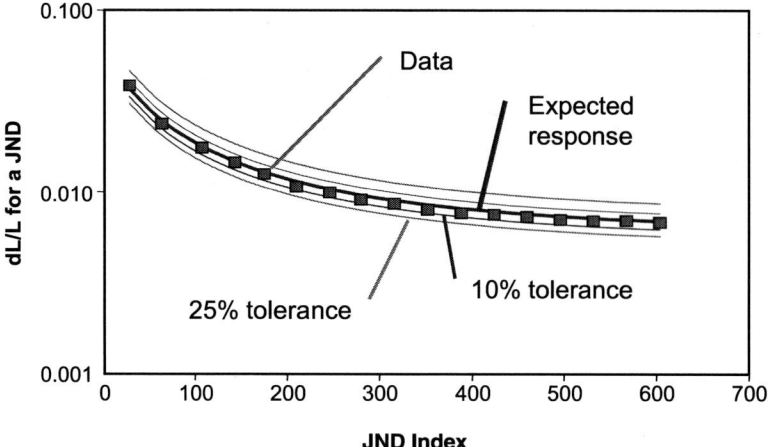

Figure 6.7 Data analysis for compliance with DICOM 3.14 GSDF showing the $\Delta L/L$ representation of the same data as a function of the JND index. The squares represent the experimentally measured data points. The thick solid line depicts the expected response for a DICOM-compliant system. The thin solid lines indicate the 10% and 25% tolerance limits. Reproduced from Ref. [12] with permission of the American Institute of Physics.

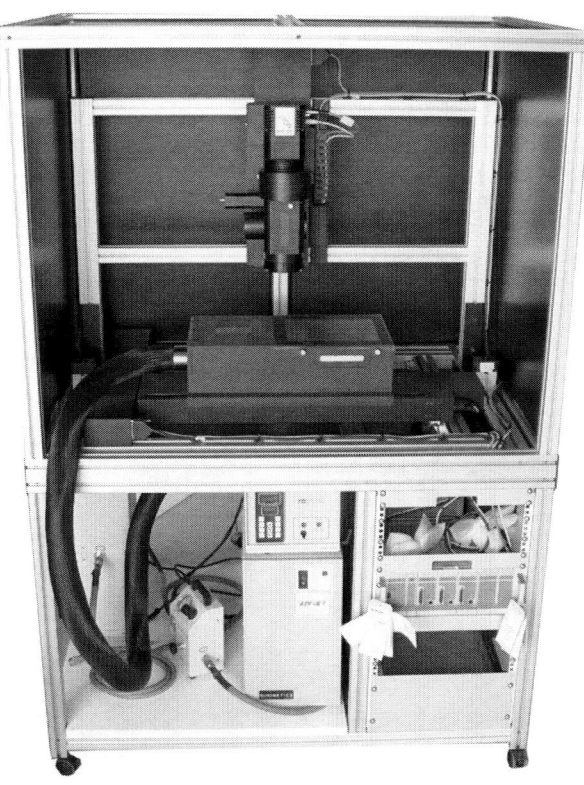

Figure 6.8 Experimental setup to measure luminance as a function of the viewing direction using Fourier optics. No rotation of the measuring device or display unit is required. Courtesy of ELectronics for Displays and IMaging devices (ELDIM), Hérouville St. Clair, France.

The second method relies on Fourier optics to map luminance intensity to angular luminance using a cooled CCD (see, for instance, Ref. [142]). The commercial system EZContrast 160D mounted on the motorized stage EZMotion (see Fig. 6.8) is manufactured by ELDIM (Hérouville St. Clair, France). This method utilizes a Fourier lens and a cooled CCD sensor. The lens provides a Fourier-transformed image of the display surface emission. Every light beam emitted from the display test area with an angle, ϕ, is focused on the focal plane at a position relative to the center of the test area that depends only on ϕ. A one-to-one correspondence exists between the direction of emission (or viewing direction) and the intensity at specific spatial locations in the imaging sensor. An optical relay system scales the Fourier transform image at the measured surface on the CCD sensor. The viewing angle map is obtained by processing the acquired image with appropriate calibration functions provided by the manufacturer. Since all of the angular information is obtained by a single imaging sensor through the Fourier lens, no rotation of the measuring device or display unit is required, nor movement of the measuring device or display monitor.

6.2 Contrast Ratio

The contrast ratio of display devices is a fundamental property to be measured. Contrast ratio is a figure that has different meanings in different communities. For instance, in the LC display industry, contrast ratio means the ratio between the maximum and minimum luminance coming out of the display when the whole screen is set to a uniform brightness. This ratio is also known elsewhere and in this book as the luminance ratio. A wide range of information can be extracted if, instead of measuring the contrast ratio with full-screen uniform fields, we use targets with varying sizes. The information provided by such measurements can reveal details about many display performance issues. Of particular importance is the measurement of the contrast ratio using small targets. The small-spot contrast ratio can illustrate phenomena that result in degradation of the local contrast. This section will describe in detail the use of small-spot contrast measurements to describe veiling glare in CRTs and electronic crosstalk in high-resolution AMLCDs.

6.2.1 Veiling glare

Veiling glare is a phenomenon created by optical and electronic scattering processes within a display that reduce image contrast. Details on the sources of veiling glare have been presented in Sec. 2.6. Veiling glare is found only in CRTs, and can be reduced by AR coatings and by absorbers in the face-plate glass.

To quantify veiling glare, we define the veiling glare ratio, G, as the bright field luminance (L_W) over the dark-spot luminance (L_D) for a 1-cm black spot on a 20-cm white circle. The calculation of G also involves the background luminance that exists in the dark-spot location with the display device in the off state:

$$G = \frac{L_D - L_B}{L_W - L_B}, \qquad (6.2)$$

where L_B is the background luminance.

Veiling glare can be measured using a telescopic luminance meter with a conic mask made out of glossy plastic or absorptive plastic films. More precisely, the veiling glare ratio can be measured using a collimated conic probe specially designed for this purpose.[8] Table 6.3 presents the measured G for a variety of CRTs obtained using a collimated conic probe. The spot size used in all measurements was 1 cm.

Advanced veiling glare measurements require the measurement of G as a function of the dark-spot radius with a low-flare luminance measurement probe. The ring response function (RRF), which is expressed by $R(r)$, is the luminance of the dark spot caused by a ring of light (see Fig. 6.9). It is computed by differentiation of the glare ratios for varying spot sizes as follows,

$$R^i(r) = \frac{\Delta(1/G_i)}{\Delta r},\qquad(6.3)$$

since, by definition,

$$1/G_i - 1/G_{i+1} = \int_{r_i}^{r_{i+1}} R(r)dr.\qquad(6.4)$$

Table 6.3 Measured G for medical and graphic arts workstation monitors.[a]

Monitor Type	G
Monochrome CRT (DS2000, Clinton)[b]	241
Monochrome CRT (SIMOMED, Siemens)	141
Monochrome CRT (Image Systems)	102
Color CRT (DELL, Trinitron)[b]	48
Color CRT (Hitachi, shadow mask)[b]	29

[a] Adapted from Ref. [10] with permission of Elsevier.
[b] Denotes systems with AR coatings.

Dark-spot test patterns

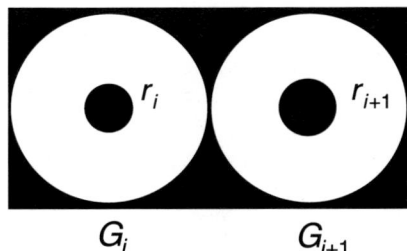

Response to luminous ring

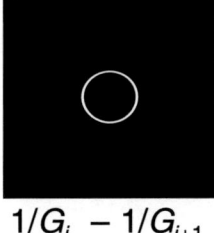

Figure 6.9 Schematic representation of the method to measure the RRF using consecutive dark-spot patterns with varying radii.

The conic probe used for these measurements has multiple baffles, a 9-mm entrance aperture, 4-mm baffle apertures, and black anodized exterior surfaces with flat black interior walls (see Fig. 6.10 for details and dimensions). In Fig. 6.11, we show the typical setup used for measurements of veiling glare in CRTs. The method, described in Ref. [8], allows a comparison of the spatial extent of the veiling glare process in different CRTs (see Fig. 6.12).

Veiling glare can be visually assessed by estimating the visibility of low-contrast targets in a 1-cm diameter dark region with and without a 20-cm diameter surrounding bright region. A flat or conic mask should be used to shield the eye from its own veiling glare or the visual response will equilibrate to a high brightness, and response in the dark spot will be diminished.

The exact relationship between a glare ratio value for a specific dark-spot size and diagnostically important degradation of medical images is not known. As a first approximation, we can expect to use CRT monitors with a G greater than 400 for primary displays and greater than 150 for secondary displays. It is important to note that veiling glare is one of the most important factors to consider when evaluating differences between color and monochrome CRTs, as clearly seen from the measured ratios shown in Table 6.3.

6.2.2 Electronic crosstalk

An undesired scene-dependent artifact is associated with an unwanted modification of the voltage effectively applied to the LC cell. The changes in pixel voltage translate into changes in light transmission through the LC, affecting the desired pixel luminance. Sources of crosstalk include incomplete pixel charging, leakage and photo-generated currents in the TFT, and parasitic capacitive coupling. Display crosstalk is more important for large-size panels having a higher resolution and gray scale. Several authors have studied crosstalk artifacts in large AM arrays and have proposed modified driving techniques that compensate for the signal distortion.[89, 108, 109] Others have focused their work on the study of the pixel voltage changes and their affect on transmission-voltage characteristics of the LC cell.[166] Although having different origins, crosstalk artifacts also have been studied for passive matrix OLEDs (PMOLEDs).[33]

In the VESA Flat Panel Display Measurements Standard,[58] methods to quantify display crosstalk are included in the gray-scale artifacts section along with other related phenomena such as streaking, ghosting, and trailing. Crosstalk is defined as "unwanted coupling between adjacent or nearby circuits that causes signal properties of one element to be injected into other elements." The standard suggests a classification into short- and long-range crosstalk effects. The complete characterization of electronic crosstalk in FPDs with high quality for medical imaging applications requires the measurement of the small-spot luminance in backgrounds of different intensity. The electronic crosstalk artifact is similar to veiling glare in CRTs since both cause contrast reduction. However, crosstalk in

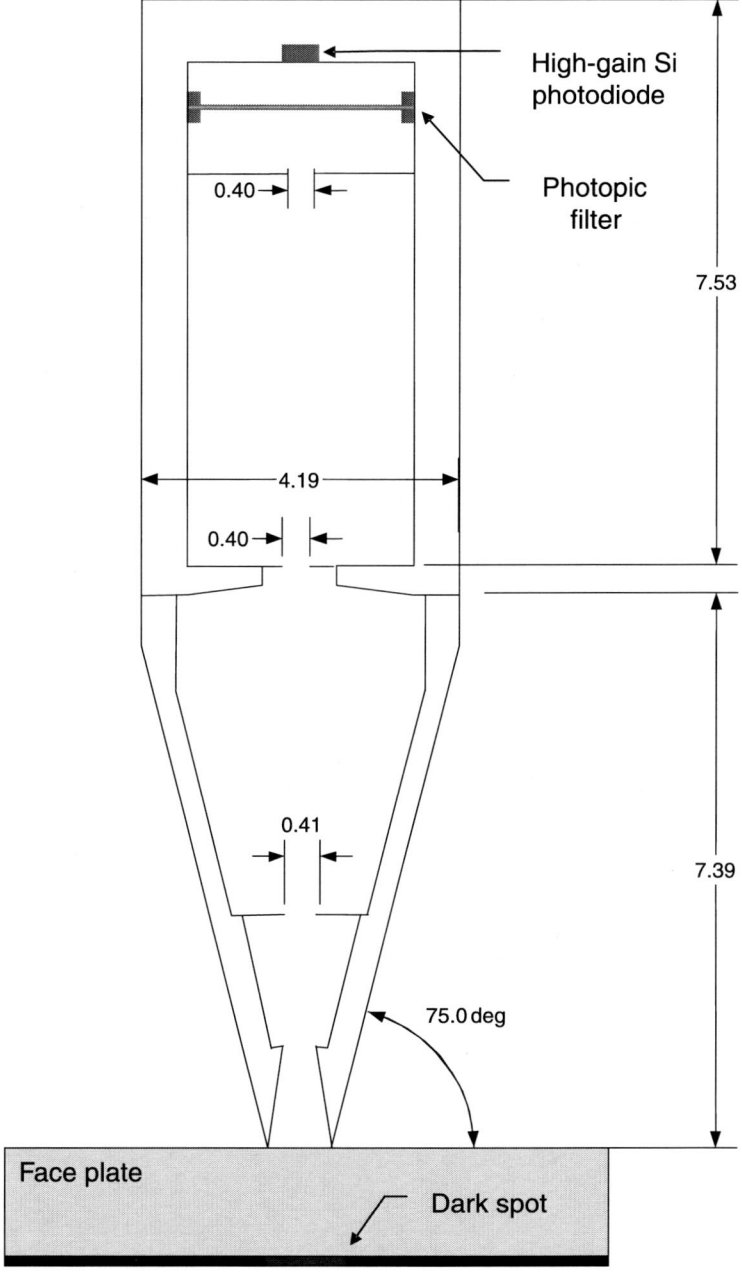

Figure 6.10 Schematic drawing of the conic collimated probe designed for measurements of veiling glare.

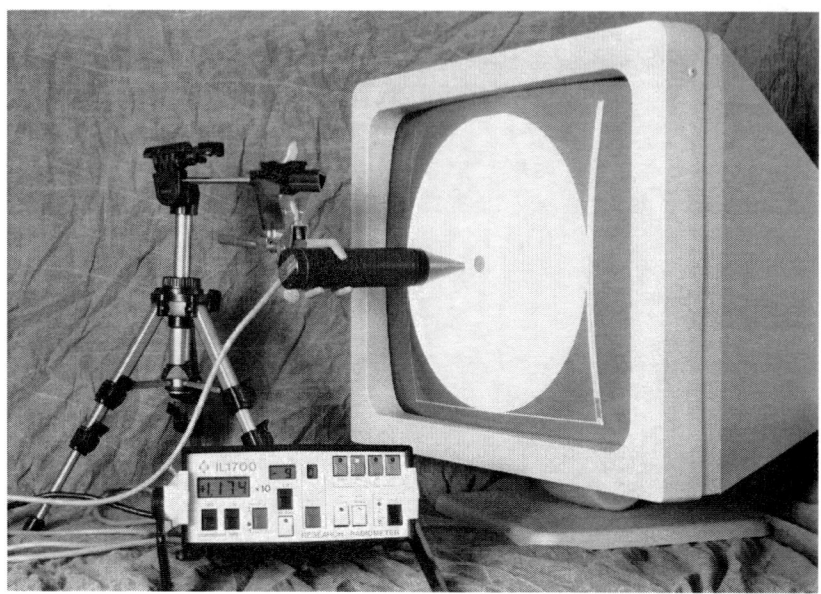

Figure 6.11 Experimental setup for measuring veiling glare. The collimated probe readings are taken by a research radiometer that connects to a computer via a serial interface. Reprinted from Ref. [60] with permission of SCAR.

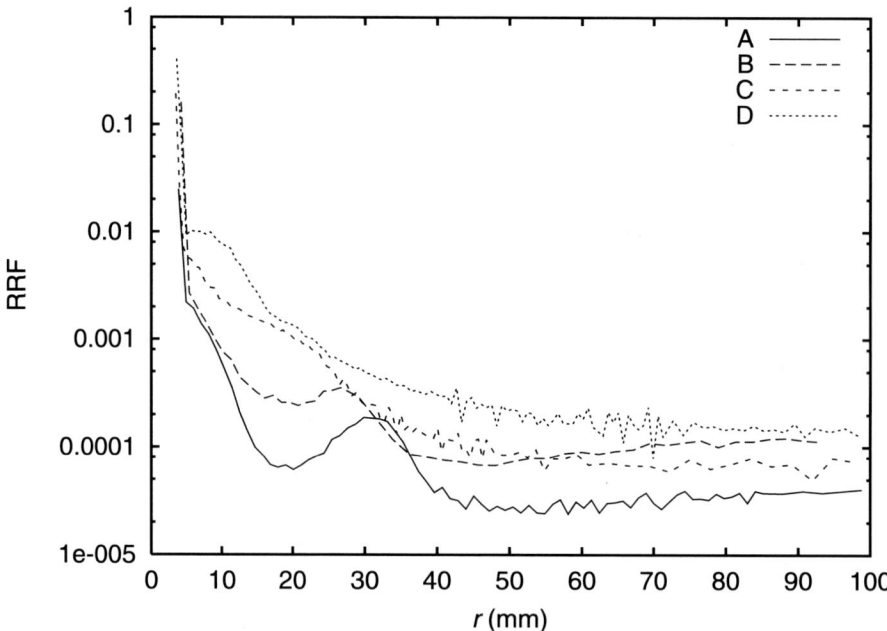

Figure 6.12 The RRF of four CRTs, where *r* is the distance from the center of the pattern: A and B are monochrome monitors for medical imaging, and C and D are color monitors. Reprinted from Ref. [10] with permission of Elsevier.

AMLCDs presents a substantial difference with respect to veiling glare: the effect of crosstalk is not rotationally symmetric due to the matrix arrangement of the display circuitry. The effect is not shift-invariant since leakage and parasitic capacitance are not uniform across the display pixel matrix. Furthermore, the crosstalk artifact cannot be treated as linear with respect to the background intensity. We have proposed[15] to evaluate the electronic crosstalk artifact by studying the change in luminance of a centered dark bar target as its width increases while the background remains at L_{max}. This approach allows end users who don't have access to the device circuits and drivers to evaluate the magnitude of the crosstalk effect in AMLCD monitors.

In a recent work,[11] measurements of display crosstalk were performed on AMLCDs using patterns consisting of a small square target of about 1 cm surrounded by a uniform luminance field (see Figs. 6.13a and 6.13b). It was found that the maximum change in target luminance associated with a change in background luminance was 1%, corresponding to a centered white target in a uniform field at an intermediate gray level. However, the measured data provided no information regarding the spatial extent of the crosstalk artifact. In more recent work,[15] Badano et al. introduced a response function that describes the magnitude and spatial profile of the one-dimensional contribution to the target luminance caused by crosstalk.

The derivation of the response function, C, is similar to the analytical model of veiling glare described in Ref. [11]. Let us define the luminance at the center of the bar target, when the bar width ($2w_d$) is equal to the screen width, as L_0. In an ideal display,[*] the luminance of the bar remains constant and equal to L_0, independently of w_d. In a real device, the luminance in the bar changes due to crosstalk from bright regions outside the target. Since the target luminance corresponds to the display L_{min}, we expect an increase in luminance for both normally white and normally black displays. The response function for crosstalk, $C(w)$, represents the differential contribution of a bright line in either the horizontal or the vertical direction to the luminance at the center of the screen. C is measured indirectly by performing a discrete summation on the experimental data for bars of different widths. We can associate two measurements with different bar widths, $L_1(w_1)$ and $L_2(w_2)$, to calculate C_{12}, the discrete crosstalk response for a line at $(w_1 + w_2)/2$. Since $C(w)$ is slowly varying, we use this expression to numerically estimate $C(w)$ from a full set of measurements of L_i (for i varying from 0 to w_{max}):

$$L_1 - L_2 = AL_0 \left[\int_{w_1}^{w_{max}} C(w)dw - \int_{w_2}^{w_{max}} C(w)dw \right] \qquad (6.5)$$

---

[*] In this context, an ideal display is defined as a display having no electronic crosstalk and no other artifact that would alter the desired pixel luminance.

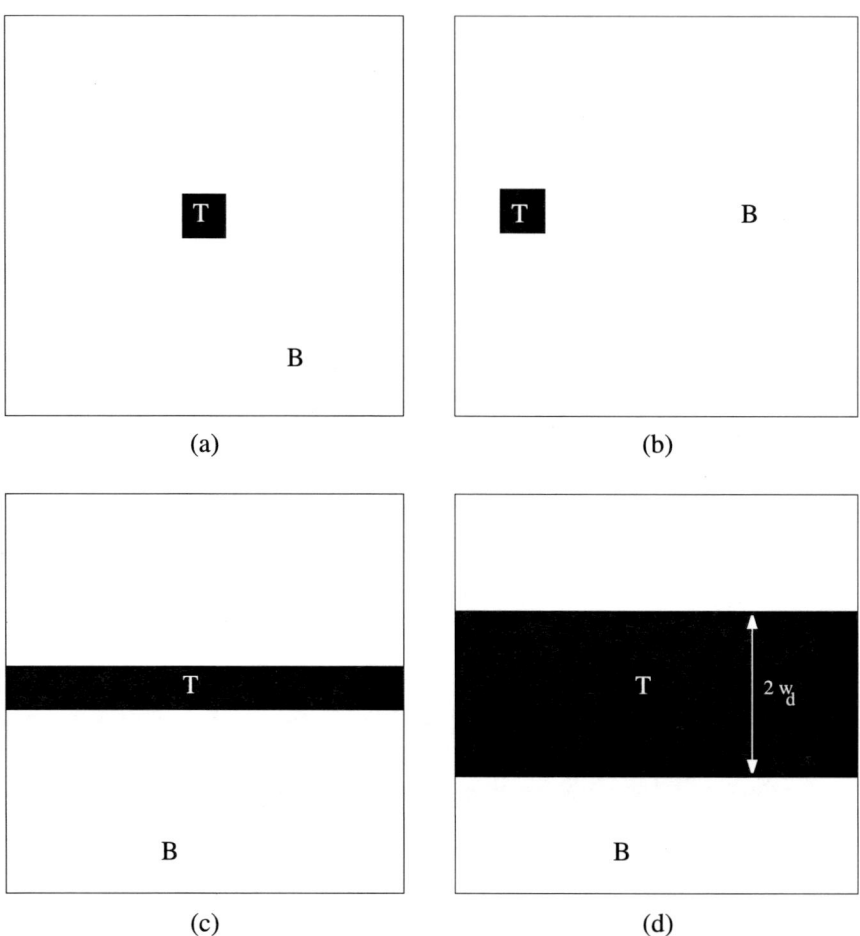

Figure 6.13 Test patterns for crosstalk measurements. Figures (a) and (b) represent patterns used in Ref. [13] with uniform background and horizontal bar. The target (T) and background (B) were assigned six luminance levels from minimum to maximum. Figures (c) and (d) are examples of the new test patterns used in this work, where the bar at a minimum luminance (T) increases its width ($2w_d$) sequentially. The background (B) is kept at maximum luminance. Reprinted from Ref. [10] with permission of Elsevier.

and

$$L_1 - L_2 \sim AL_0 C_{12}(w_2 - w_1). \tag{6.6}$$

Under the assumption that C is constant within a small change in bar width (i.e., $w_1 \sim w_2$), we can compute the crosstalk response function as follows:

$$C_{12} \sim \frac{L_1 - L_2}{AL_0(w_2 - w_1)} . \tag{6.7}$$

Figure 6.14 shows the response functions in the horizontal and vertical directions for two AMLCDs: LCD1 and LCD2. In the case of LCD1, the magnitude of the crosstalk is low at distances larger than 10 mm approaching levels on the order of 10^{-5}–10^{-6}. At 10 mm, the crosstalk effect is on the order of 10^{-5}. We note a difference in the tails of the horizontal and vertical response functions. The horizontal crosstalk peaks at about 6 mm and decreases to 10^{-6} at about 15 mm, while the vertical response decreases monotonically to 5×10^{-6}. This difference in final values of $C(w)$ could be attributed to the 16:10 aspect ratio of the monitor LCD1. For this monitor, the horizontal crosstalk is five times larger than the vertical crosstalk at large w_d.

For LCD2, the horizontal and vertical $C(w)$ values converged to a value of 5×10^{-6}. Data for w less than 3 mm should not be interpreted as crosstalk since the signal comes from a target that is smaller than the effective field of view of the probe. We can estimate the luminance gain in the centered dark bar using the response functions $C(w)$ for any given test pattern consisting of a dark target and a bright surrounding field. For instance, for a 1-cm bar in a screen with a width of 31 cm, the relative luminance gain is given by

$$\frac{L_c}{L_0} = 2 \int_{5 \text{ mm}}^{150 \text{ mm}} C(w)\,dw \sim 2(150 - 5)C', \qquad (6.8)$$

where C' is the asymptotic limit of $C(w)$ for $w_d > 10$ mm. For LCD1, L_c/L_0 is about 0.0015 for a vertical bar and 0.0006 for a horizontal bar. For LCD2, both vertical and horizontal bars will be affected equally with a gain of about 0.0015. If we consider that the gains due to horizontal and vertical crosstalk are independent and can be added together to obtain the gain in luminance for a small square target,[*] we find that the relative increase in luminance is on the order of 0.42% for LCD1 and 0.60% for LCD2 for a dark target in a background at L_{max}. The analysis of the crosstalk effect using the response function $C(w)$ reflects similar magnitudes of the luminance change obtained for square targets using the same photopic probe. The function $C(w)$ also provides insight into the spatial profile of the contribution to the target luminance variation. Further investigations are still needed to determine if the measured short-range crosstalk is due to electronic phenomena, or instead is associated with local scattering of light in a thin transparent face plate, sometimes called halation (as suggested in Ref. [9]). Martin et al.[115] investigated crosstalk effects using test patterns with off-center square targets and horizontal half bars. They showed that for high-resolution AMLCDs, the effect of the left and right half bars is not symmetrical: the effect of a left half bar increases with the distance between the target and the left panel edge. Their results suggest that crosstalk effects depend essentially on the length of the horizontal half bars, and that crosstalk is at its maximum along the horizontal direction of portrait-mode displays for dark targets in bright backgrounds.

---

[*] Note that this assumption does not imply that $C(w)$ is linear with respect to I_o.

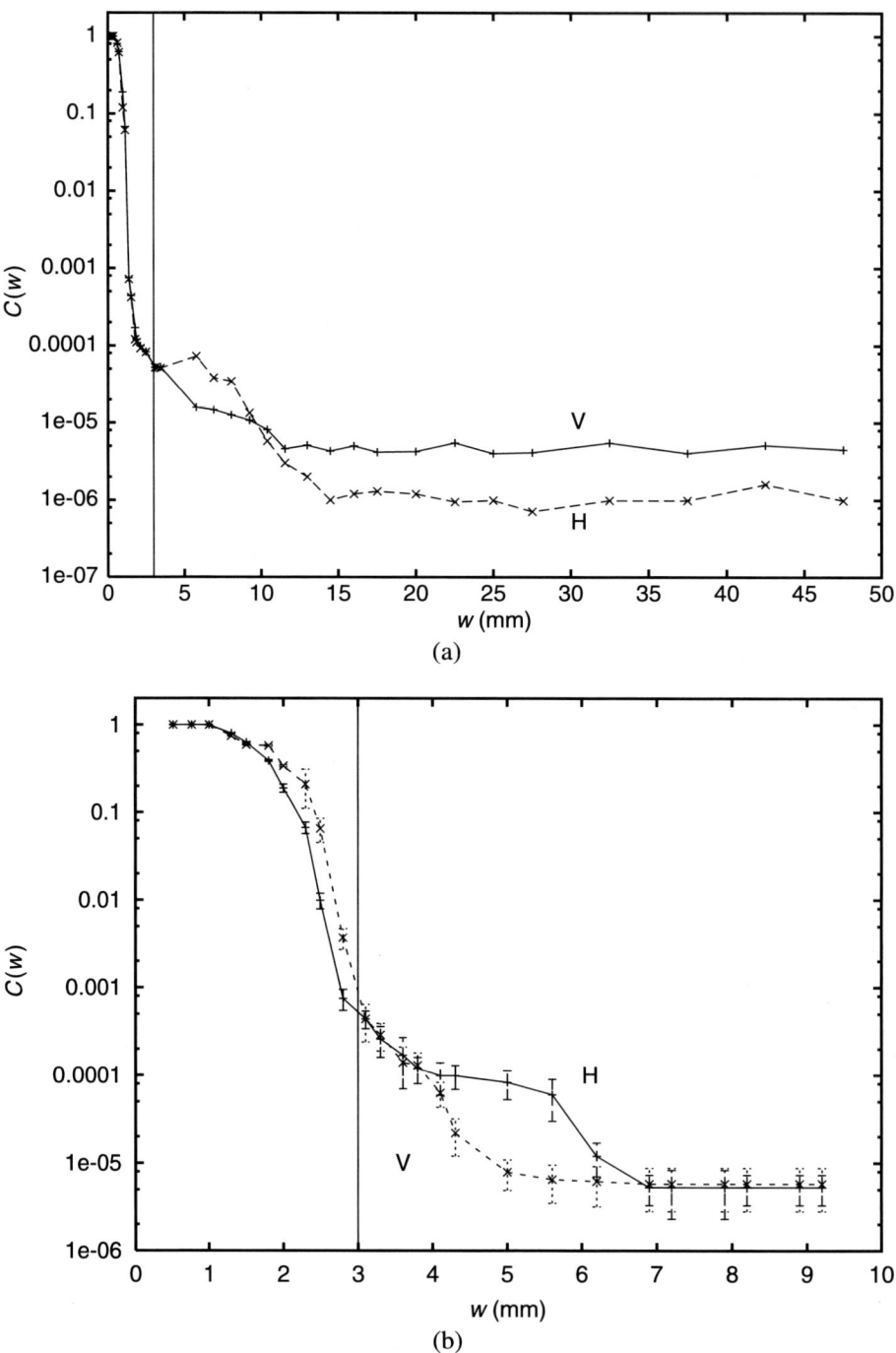

Figure 6.14   Crosstalk response functions $C(w)$ for LCD1 (a) and LCD2 (b) for a horizontal bar (H) and a vertical bar (V). The line at 3 mm indicates the minimum bar width that the method can measure due primarily to the field of view of the collimated luminance probe. Adapted from Ref. [15].

6.3 Spatial Frequency

High-resolution digital radiographs can effectively record the detail of high-contrast structures. The sharpness of these details is contained in high spatial frequencies. Medical image CRT displays have formats of 1 k, 1.5 k, or 2 k pixels along one of the pixel array dimensions, which corresponds to about a 0.15–0.30-mm nominal pixel size. In CRTs, pixels are circular with a near-Gaussian profile that is nonisotropic, location-dependent, and luminance-dependent (see Fig. 6.15). The addressable pixel size should be as close as possible to the actual pixel size to deliver the desired resolution. This is depicted in the resolution-to-addressability ratio (RAR), which is given by the pixel FWHM over the pixel nominal size. It was shown by Muka et al. that an RAR between 0.9–1.1 provides the best display of medical radiographs.[124]

The resolution response of CRTs degrades over time due to a deterioration of the electron optics, and most importantly, by an increase in the beam current's compensation of the luminance reduction due to aging of the phosphor. Conventional methods evaluate resolution by measuring a spread function from either point, line, or edge patterns and then computing the modulation transfer function (MTF). CRT devices vary significantly in resolution as a function of position and brightness. Therefore, conventional linear analysis of high-contrast test images cannot be used. Blur associated with the electron beam current and with light diffusion linearly modifies the luminance of an image. However, visual perception is proportional to log-luminance, which is roughly proportional to display value, and therefore the

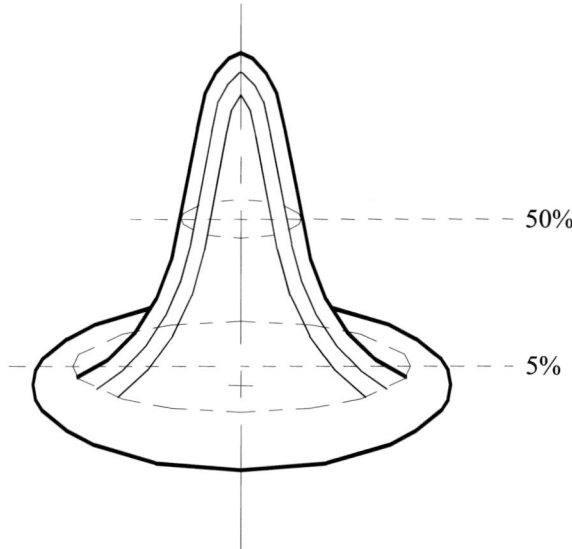

Figure 6.15 Typical profile of a CRT beam spot indicating the 50% and 5% widths. Reprinted from Ref. [46] with permission of K. Compton.

beam current increases exponentially with display value (i.e., displays are nonlinear devices). Additionally, the spot size is strongly dependent on the beam current, making blur a function of position (i.e., CRTs are nonstationary devices).

All advanced methods for characterizing the resolution properties of display systems are based on Fourier analysis of a recorded image of the output luminance pattern. For instance, investigators have proposed the use of a figure of merit based on the integral of the MTF up to a given limit frequency (sometimes associated with the limiting frequency response of the human visual system). Since this class of methods incorporates psychophysics elements into a figure of merit, it has been used to predict perceptual visual quality.[19, 21] An alternative to this method is to adjust the MTF with a filter function to match the response of human vision.

The methods used to evaluate the MTF from high-contrast lines or edges require linear signals and a stationary response. Therefore, linear systems analysis is not appropriate for evaluating the resolution of a display (particularly for CRTs) as it relates to visual performance.

The measurement of the resolution response using linear analysis methods can be made only when the signal changes are restricted to sufficiently small values such that the signal response can be considered locally linear. A CCD camera with a macro lens can be used to record test patterns with high magnification. The camera should have at least 10 bits of signal range or have features permitting a high-contrast camera response. Since the resolution is reduced to a relative result (the MTF), the specific gamma response of the display does not need to be known. The resolution of the display can also be a function of orientation. This is shown in Fig. 6.16, which presents horizontal and vertical MTFs for a monochrome CRT.

To determine the resolution properties of display devices, two methods can be used. The MTF can be obtained by measuring a line-spread function and performing a one-dimensional Fourier analysis. The second method involves displaying artificial white noise images and recording the response of the display.[14, 165] A two-dimensional Fourier analysis is then performed over multiple blocks to get an estimate of the signal power spectrum. The MTF is computed as the modulus of the Fourier transform. Since only the frequency profile is needed, no scaling is required for the power spectrum calculations.

The resolution properties of a display device can be assessed visually without the need for expensive instrumentation. Using a "CX" pattern,[102] observers can determine the degree of blur present in different screen locations. This technique has been successfully incorporated in quality control patterns. As general criteria, the MTF of primary displays needs to be larger than 35% at the Nyquist frequency, while secondary displays require 25%.

A methodology for the assessment of the MTF characteristics of display devices using a photographic-grade CCD camera was introduced by Samei et al.[144] In this method, the linearization of the CCD signal was achieved with a sequence of photographs of targets at different luminance levels. The main advantage of the method is that the instrumentation is portable and can be performed in a clinical environment.

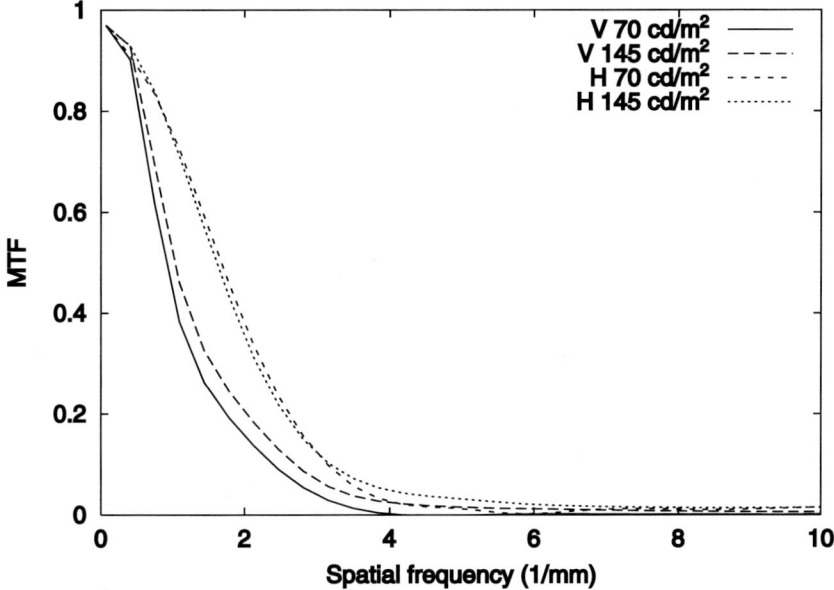

Figure 6.16 Measured MTFs of a P45 CRT at two luminance levels and at two orientations. The MTF in the direction parallel to the scan raster lines (H) is larger than the MTF in the perpendicular direction (V). Adapted from Ref. [14].

In AMLCDs, the resolution is dependent on the orientation of the signal with respect to the pixel matrix due to the discrete array of approximately rectangular pixels. The pixel structure and its aperture ratio determine a different fixed pattern that has to be taken into account when measuring the display's resolution characteristics. Table 6.4 presents a brief list of fundamental technological differences between CRTs and AMLCDs. Of those, the most important factor with respect to resolution is the pixel structure.

Often, measurement methods in the spatial and frequency domains do not provide consistent results between or within technologies.[14] The MTF values obtained using the broadband response and line pattern methods do not agree for AMLCDs due to the effect of nonstochastic residuals. The same effect is seen in noise estimates that rely on image variance or on noise power spectrum (NPS) calculations, as discussed in the next section.

6.4 Noise

Noise sources in a display device can be catalogued in different ways (see Table 6.4). For instance, we can discriminate sources of spatial noise (i.e., CRT phosphor granularity) versus sources of temporal noise (image lag in AMLCDs). However, when performing measurements of display performance and using displays for visual tasks, the boundaries between spatial and temporal noise become blurred by the

Table 6.4 Fundamental technological differences between CRTs and AMLCDs.

Property	CRT	AMLCD
Mechanism	Light-emitting	Light-modulating
Front panel	Curved	Flat
Array formation	Scanning beam	AM addressing
Emission	Near-Lambertian	Far from Lambertian
Long-range interactions	Veiling glare	Crosstalk
Pixel structure	Gaussian spot	Rectangular (subpixel domains)
Noise	Phosphor noise	LC variations Cell thickness variations Spacers
Structured noise	Raster	Inactive pixel regions
Artifacts	Deflection Landing	Cell voltage variation Backlight nonuniformity
Temporal	Flicker	Flicker and LC ghosting

integration time of the observer or of the instrumentation. Assessing temporal noise sources requires a system capable of responding at a faster rate than the refresh rate of the display device in a synchronized mode. Generally temporal noise is dominant in the low-luminance regions, while spatial noise created by the phosphor granularity in CRTs is dominant in the mid- and high-luminance regions.

Spatial noise in a display device can obscure small, low-contrast image features. This is analogous to the effect of x-ray quantum noise in CT and radiography. It is useful to employ a 10x magnifier to view the light-emission pattern from a region with a uniform, mid-gray brightness level. A variety of noise patterns will be seen in CRT devices in addition to the expected raster lines. The digital photographs in Fig. 6.17 were obtained from uniform gray images.

Roberts et al. studied a method to measure static noise using a stray-light elimination probe.[140] They found that for large signal variations, an imaging device (i.e., a CCD camera) did not measure noise accurately due to flare in the lens. However, display spatial noise is always associated with small signal variations. In this case, Fourier methods can be used to determine the noise correlation properties. Estimation of the NPS involves CCD camera recordings of a small, uniform field and two-dimensional Fourier analysis to obtain the NPS. As shown in Fig. 6.18, single-crystal phosphors (P45) have less power (i.e., are less noisy) than blended, multiple-crystal phosphors (P104). The magnitude of the NPS estimation is on the same order of magnitude as the NPS of a computed radiography

Figure 6.17 Photographs of CRT screens using a macro lens. From left to right: a color monitor screen with its RGB dots in a delta arrangement, a P104 screen showing high granularity, and a P45 screen.

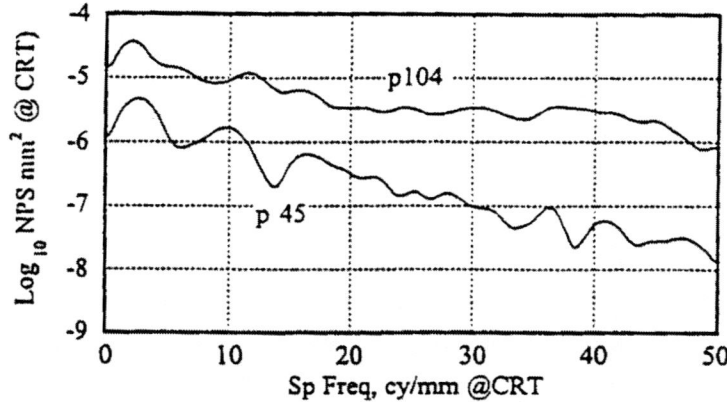

Figure 6.18 NPS measurements for P104 and P45 CRT phosphors. Reprinted from Ref. [124].

image at an exposure of 1 mR. The NPS profiles of CRTs can have higher magnitudes in the high spatial frequencies because of phosphor granularity.

Another way to characterize noise associated with spatial variations of luminance is to compute the luminance variations in images of uniform fields. The luminance noise (LN) is then expressed as a percentage with respect to the mean value.

Recently, Badano et al. showed that methods to measure luminance noise are affected by the details of the pixel design (see Fig. 6.19).[7] Because of the subpixel structures present in FPDs, noise estimates based on image variance and absolute magnitude of the power spectrum decrease with increasing aperture sizes of the recording device (for instance, a CCD camera) until reaching an asymptotic value for aperture sizes larger than the display pixel dimensions.

Another recent contribution to this problem is the use of apertures to remove the effects of the subpixel structure. Figure 6.20 presents preliminary results regarding the use of two types of apertures: a sliding circular (SC) aperture and a pixel-aligned (PA) aperture. The PA aperture averages the luminance field within the pixel and

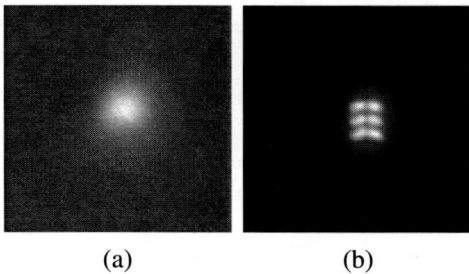

(a)   (b)

Figure 6.19 Single-pixel images of a CRT (a) and an AMLCD (b). The Gaussian luminance map corresponding to the CRT electron beam spot contrasts with the six sharply defined subpixel regions in a chevron arrangement (due to three color strips and two domains with different director orientations). Adapted from Ref. [14].

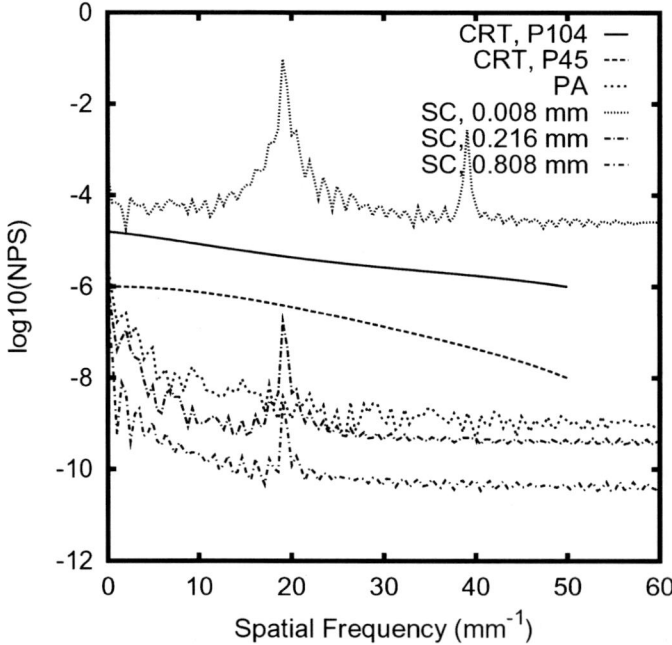

Figure 6.20 NPS measurements for AMLCDs and CRTs using apertures. The NPS of the high-resolution AMLCD was taken using a scientific low-noise CCD camera with a 1300 × 1340 element array (at 18 CCD pixels per FPD pixel width). The NPS of the CRT was taken from Ref. [124]. In the graph, PA represents pixel-aligned aperture and SC stands for sliding circular aperture. See text for details.

therefore leaves in the image the components of luminance noise associated with interpixel variations (as opposed to intrapixel variations caused by the subpixel structure). The figure shows that when measured under high resolution, the noise of an AMLCD with highly structured pixels results in overestimation of the perceived noise level. The application of a PA aperture yields noise estimates that are below CRT noise levels and more consistent with perceived noise. For more details, see Ref. [7].

6.5 Reflectance

Due to the nature of CRT emissive structures, a large fraction of the light that illuminates the device is reflected either at the front surface or after multiple internal scattering. A rough front surface cannot be used because it will introduce image blur due to the thick glass face plate. Light that enters the face plate and strikes the phosphor layer encounters a structure that, by design, is highly reflective. The phosphor structure consists of small grains in a binder with a reflective backing. Similar to radiographic screens, this structure is designed for good light emission with little self-absorption. Therefore, monochrome CRT devices used for high-resolution radiographic display typically exhibit poor performance with respect to both specular and diffuse reflection of ambient light. This has forced the use of very dark rooms for diagnostic interpretation and has severely handicapped the deployment of electronic imaging systems into patient care areas.

To dampen specular reflections, AR structures are used that consist of several thin-film layers designed to reduce the reflectance of the front surface by increasing the light transmission into the face plate.[157] Normally, AR coatings will also include a conductive layer that dissipates the static charge generated at the front surface and helps maintain a dust-free surface.[133] The reflections from AR coatings can shift colors when illuminated with a broad-spectrum light source because of the wavelength dependency of the thin-film response.[31] However, by decreasing the reflection of incident light, AR coatings may increase diffuse reflections since more light enters the face plate. The effectiveness of AR coatings is then associated with a compromise between the specular and diffuse components of ambient light reflection.

To reduce diffuse reflectance, CRTs may have an absorptive face plate that attenuates and scatters light several times in the glass. For a face plate with a transmittance of 50%, the diffuse reflections will be reduced by at least 25% because the reflected light will travel through the glass twice. More reduction is typically found because of the oblique directions that the reflected light may travel and because of multiple internal scattering. However, this reduction comes at the expense of a 50% decrease in display brightness. In color monitors, the black matrix material that is between phosphor dots is of considerable benefit in absorbing incident light without reducing brightness. In this sense, the design of color monitors is advantageous from the standpoint of both veiling glare and ambient reflection. However, to date black matrix phosphor technologies have not been used with high-brightness monochrome phosphors.

Ideally, a display device will be designed specifically to absorb ambient light. New FPD devices offer opportunities for the absorption of ambient light that is not possible with CRTs, and AMLCDs are being designed to optimize the absorption of ambient light for use in sunlit environments, such as for avionic applications.[34]

The reflectance of display devices can be characterized by separate components involving specular and diffuse light scattering. Both components have markedly distinct effects on image quality and require different experimental measurement methods.

6.5.1 Reflectance models

Specular reflections produce distinct virtual images at the display surface that mirror luminous objects in the room. The reflected luminance, $L_S(\theta)$, can be related to the source luminance, $L_s(\theta)$, by

$$R_S(\theta) = L_S(\theta)/L_s(\theta) \ ,$$

where θ is the incident angle and R_S is the dimensionless specular reflection coefficient. Specular reflections can severely degrade image quality in specific regions by adding interfering structured signals to the image content and by reducing contrast in localized regions.

Ambient illumination of the display surface will also produce diffuse reflections with no detail and similar intensity over the entire screen. Typically, light photons will strike the display surface and emerge with a broad angular distribution due to surface roughness and multiple scattering processes. Diffuse reflections (R_D) can be characterized by a coefficient defined as

$$R_D(\theta_i, \phi_i, \theta_o, \phi_o) = L_D(\theta_o, \phi_o)/I(\theta_i, \phi_i) \ , \tag{6.9}$$

where $L_D(\theta_o, \phi_o)$ is the diffusely reflected luminance measured at an angle (θ_o, ϕ_o) from the surface normal, and $I(\theta_i, \phi_i)$ is the illuminance at the surface from light incident at an angle (θ_i, ϕ_i). Because of the units associated with measures of luminance (nit) and illuminance (lux), R_D has units of 1/sr. For an ideal Lambertian reflector, L_D is independent of the angle and the reflection coefficient is only a function of the illumination angle, $R_D(\theta_i, \phi_i)$. If the illumination of the surface is from many directions, as is the case in a room, the illuminance will have differential contributions from different directions such that

$$I = \int_0^{2\pi} \int_0^{\frac{\pi}{2}} I(\theta_i, \phi_i) d\theta_i d\phi_i, \tag{6.10}$$

where $I(\theta_i, \phi_i)d\theta_i d\phi_i$ is the differential illuminance averaged over all angles. The diffuse reflection coefficient that is specific to a particular lighting condition can be defined as

$$R_D(\theta_o) = L_D(\theta_o)/I \ ,$$

where $R_D(\theta_o)$ is a weighted average that depends on the angular distribution of illumination.

6.5.2 Measuring display reflections

Methods for measuring reflection coefficients have been the focus of recent research efforts.[24, 90, 112, 113] While test methods have been proposed as part of an international standard,[87] the defined experimental techniques are deficient with respect to repeatability and reliability due to variations in instrumentation response and light source geometry.[160] Moreover, Kelley[97] and Becker[24] have recently suggested that difficulties can arise for FPD devices when reflections fall in the intermediate regime between specular and diffuse reflections. They propose using the bidirectional reflection distribution function (BRDF) to fully describe the performance in any ambient lighting condition [similar to Eq. (6.9)]. The BRDF is the luminance reflected from a display at all angles for a given illumination condition; it is a function of both source direction and type, and of the observer's viewing direction. See Sec. 6.5.3 for more information.

We used an application-oriented method[4] to experimentally evaluate diffuse and specular reflection coefficients from display devices that are representative of the current state-of-the-art for medical imaging purposes (manufactured by Clinton Electronics Corp., Siemens AG, Image Systems Corp., and Data Ray Corp.), along with a color monitor (manufactured by Hitachi Ltd.). We also included measurements for radiographic film (manufactured by Eastman Kodak and Ekstascan HNC) and for AMLCDs of current design (manufactured by Hosiden Corp. and Optical Imaging Systems Inc.).

For the measurement of specular reflection, a small uniform source of light creates a specularly reflected image on an otherwise black display surface located in a dark room. To minimize the diffuse component, the area of the light source must be as small as possible. We used a small spot lamp with a diffuse white luminous area of about a 5.7-cm diameter (see Fig. 6.21). Using a spot photometer, the luminance of the reflected image is then related to the luminance of the light source when viewed directly. We used a Minolta LS110 spot photometer that measures luminance in a one-third deg spot. Typical values for the reflection angles include 15 deg and 30 deg at distances ranging from 50 to 100 cm. Since most displays are viewed from a direction near the surface normal, we made measure-

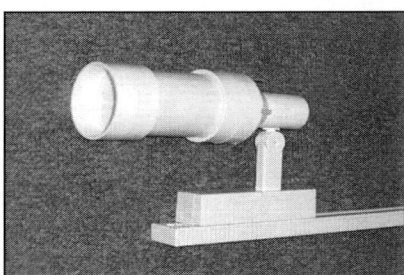

Figure 6.21   Small spot lamp used as a light source for specular reflections. The diameter of the light fixture is about 5 cm.

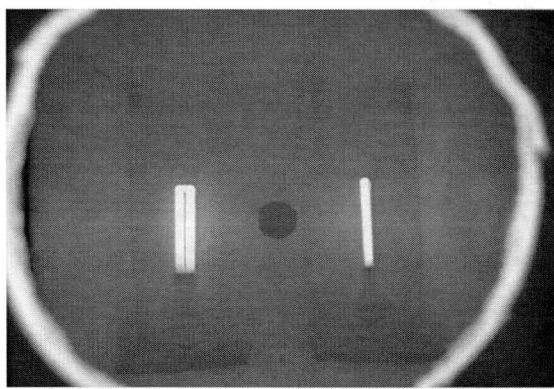

Figure 6.22 Portable white room viewed in a normal direction through a hole in the back of the box.

ments with the light source and the spot photometer at 75 cm from the center of the display and 15 deg from the surface normal.

The diffuse reflection from display devices is measured by illuminating the display device in an off condition with a diffuse source.* Others have used various lamps at different positions in a dark room.[87, 160] Inconsistent results can be caused in part by variations in illumination that come from the walls, objects, and persons in the room. Therefore, to establish consistent illumination conditions, we used a reproducible, portable device consisting of a 40 x 40 x 40-cm box with white reflective sides and two 9-W fluorescent lamps located at the back corners to create a "white box." Illuminance was measured with a small illuminance probe (International Light, Inc., IL 1400) placed on the surface of the display. In such a white box, luminance in a normal direction with respect to the display surface is measured through a hole in the back of the box with a spot photometer. The absence of specular reflections is confirmed by the dark circle that appears in the display surface when viewed through the back aperture (see Fig. 6.22).

The white box, shown in Fig. 6.23, in effect creates a reproducible white room that can be taken to different locations for comparison measurements, providing an angular distribution of illumination representative of that found in patient care areas. The measured luminance per illuminance, R_D, is expressed in lumens/sr/m^2 (i.e., cd/m^2 or nits) per lumens/m^2 (i.e., lux), which is measured in units of 1/sr. More conveniently, the diffuse reflection coefficient R_D is expressed in units of luminance per illuminance, since these can be directly associated with visual effects.

---

*   For devices that rely on changes in transmission to modulate the luminance of the scene (i.e., transilluminated film, LC displays), measurements of diffuse reflections with fields at different luminance levels are required.

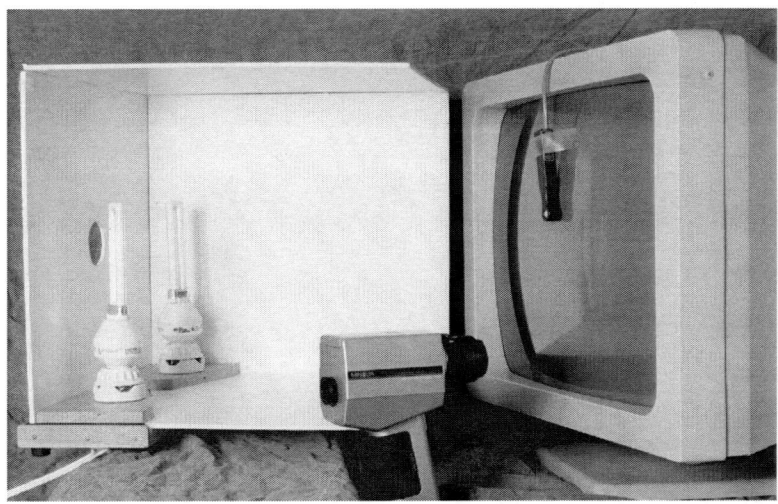

Figure 6.23 White reflective box used to measure diffuse reflection coefficients consisting of a 40 x 40 x 40-cm box with white reflective sides and two compact fluorescent lamps located at the back corners. The front side of the box has been removed for illustration purposes. Luminance is measured in a normal direction through a hole in the back of the box with a spot photometer. Illuminance is measured with a small illuminance probe placed on the surface of the display. Reprinted from Ref. [60] with permission of SCAR.

As discussed previously, the diffuse reflection coefficient is specific to the angular distribution of illumination associated with particular measurement conditions. When using the experimental technique described in this work, the obtained result corresponds to

$$R_D(0) = L_D(0)/I , \qquad (6.11)$$

where I is the total illuminance at the display surface. The illuminance probe we used records incident light with a broad angular response (International Light Inc., model SCL110).

When measuring reflections from radiographic film, attention must be given to the optical density values in the image since they affect the light diffusion characteristics of the device. For this reason, reflection measurements were taken with three films having different optical density values. The difference in values is associated, in part, with the ambient light that is transmitted to the view box and reflected back. This dependence by the reflection coefficients on the image luminance pattern is not observed in CRTs, where measurements are performed with the display turned off.

Now that practical experimental techniques have been delineated to measure specular and diffuse reflection coefficients, next the experimental results will be reported for several high-performance display devices including film, monochrome and color CRTs, and AMLCDs. The results are compared with data obtained for transilluminated radiographic film using the same experimental techniques.

Table 6.5 reports the results on diffuse and specular coefficients for all display devices studied in this work. The specular reflection coefficients varied from 0.0019 to 0.042. The coefficients measured for the monitors without an AR coating are consistent with the value computed according to Fresnel equations for a glass-air optical boundary (0.04). Devices with an AR coating have smaller specu-

Table 6.5 Reflection coefficients for high-performance display devices.

Display Type	R_S	R_D (1/sr)
Film[a]		
Radiographic film (at OD^b = 2.8)	0.013 ± 0.001	0.020 ± 0.001
Radiographic film (at OD = 1.0)	0.024 ± 0.001	–
Radiographic film (at OD = 0.1)	0.039 ± 0.001	–
Radiographic film (with chest image)	–	0.026 ± 0.001
CRT		
Monochrome CRT DS2000 HB[c]	0.0034 ± 0.0001	0.018 ± 0.001
Monochrome CRT Simomed HM54[d]	0.0055 ± 0.0001	0.031 ± 0.001
Monochrome CRT DR80(25)[e]	0.010 ± 0.001	0.064 ± 0.001
Color CRT Superscan Elite 751[f]	0.017 ± 0.001	0.025 ± 0.001
Display	R_S	R_D (1/sr)
Monochrome CRT ML24[g]	0.037 ± 0.001	0.058 ± 0.001
Monochrome CRT DR90(21)[e]	0.042 ± 0.001	0.032 ± 0.001
AMLCD		
Color AMLCD Akia 145 (black state)[h]	0.0019 ± 0.0001^i	0.024 ± 0.001
Color AMLCD Akia 145 (gray state)	0.0021 ± 0.0001^i	0.023 ± 0.001
Color AMLCD avionics (off state)[i]	–	0.005 ± 0.001^j
Monochrome AMLCD (off state)[k]	0.012 ± 0.001	0.023 ± 0.001

[a] From Eastman Kodak (Ekstascan HNC).
[b] Optical density.
[c] From Clinton Electronics Corp.
[d] From Siemens AG.
[e] From Data Ray Corp.
[f] From Hitachi Ltd.
[g] From Image Systems Corp.
[h] AMLCD panel from Hosiden Corp.
[i] From Optical Imaging Systems Inc.
[j] Display devices with AR coating.
[k] C3 from DOME Imaging Systems, Inc.

lar reflection coefficients. Among them, the lowest R_S was measured for monitors having the most advanced AR coating designs. All the specular coefficients for devices with AR coatings are smaller than those for radiographic film. The measured values for the diffuse reflection coefficients all fall within a smaller range (0.018–0.064 nits/lux) except an AMLCD designed for avionic applications. This measurement proves that low diffuse reflection coefficients can be achieved with advanced optical design. Although the values of R_D for all the other devices (including radiographic film) are comparable, the effects on image quality are more significant in those devices with low luminance. The color CRT performs better due to an AR coating and to the black matrix in the phosphor layer. Random errors are estimated from the standard deviation of 10 consecutive measurements.

6.5.3 Bidirectional reflection distribution function

For new flat-panel systems, the surface reflections include a local haze component. Results are dependent on both the input and output angles, which can be described as the bidirectional reflection distribution function (BRDF). The BRDF, a formalism often used in optics,[55] is defined for any reflecting object as the ratio of differential reflected luminance, dL_o, to the differential illuminance, dE_i, incident on the surface. In this work, we consider the reflectance from the display to be shift-invariant, or independent of position across the screen, therefore neglecting all edge-related phenomena. The complete expression is then given by the six-dimensional function

$$BRDF(\theta_i, \phi_i, \theta_o, \phi_o, \lambda, p) = \frac{dL_o(\theta_o, \phi_o, \lambda, p)}{dE_i(\theta_i, \phi_i, \lambda, p)}, \qquad (6.12)$$

where λ is the photon wavelength and p is the polarization of the incoming light beam. The BRDF is measured in units of sr^{-1}. The incidence angle of ambient light is defined by (θ_i, ϕ_i), while θ_o and ϕ_o are the angles that define the direction of reflected light.

The precise evaluation of this function is time consuming and costly. The BRDF can be measured using a goniometric setup with a fixed light source and a variable detector, with a variable source and a fixed detector, or with a conoscopic approach, where the directional intensity is mapped into a two-dimensional distribution recorded by a position-sensitive planar detector. The first two methods suffer from dependence on precise source and detector positioning, which must be less than 1 deg. The third method requires expensive instrumentation. Monte Carlo simulation methods have been used to predict the reflection properties of novel display devices.[5, 16]

The intermediate component of the reflection signature called "haze" can be characterized by taking incremental measurements of the reflected luminance

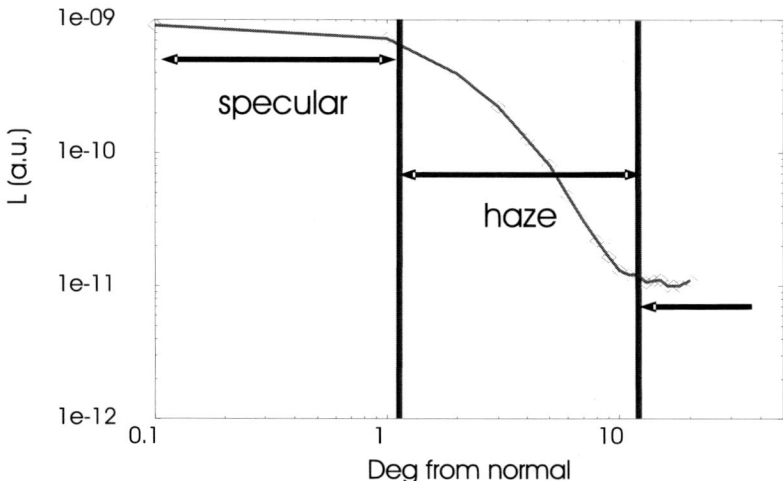

Figure 6.24 One-dimensional reflection signature of an AMLCD. The value at 0.1 deg corresponds to the measurement at 0 deg, which is within the specular window. Depending on the specific definitions used for the specular reflection, we can identify the "haze" window as expanding from 1 to 10 deg. The measurements for angles larger than 10 deg reflect the diffuse component.

obtained with a small diffuse light source (5 mm in diameter). As the angle between the direction of the measurement with the light-measuring device and the specular direction increases, we can record one slice of the full BRDF as shown in Fig. 6.24. Note that in this experiment, the uncertainties in the positioning of the source and meter were sufficient to mask the specular peak (between 0 and 1 deg).

6.6 Evaluation Software and Standards

Comprehensive tools to display test patterns in monitors and simultaneously interface with photometric equipment to capture the luminance variations from the screen are rare and typically expensive. For some of the basic measurements described in this book such as gray-scale resolution, many software tools are available from different vendors and are typically included with the light-measuring device.

A more flexible research tool that is in the public domain is DisplayTool,[59] a graphic software application for evaluating the performance of a display device. Specific performance characteristics that influence display quality are evaluated with different test patterns. DisplayTool can generate a large number of variable patterns while different light meters can be used for each performance measure. DisplayTool can also be used to compare measured performance with the requirements of specific medical applications, then tracked over time to detect performance changes. The current version includes applications to study luminance response, modulation transfer, noise, veiling glare, and contrast transfer. Display-

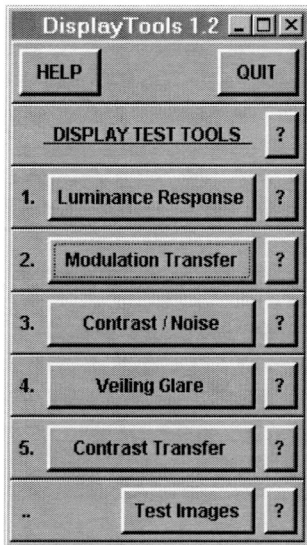

Figure 6.25 DisplayTool opening window. Each button starts a graphic test for a specific display quality factor.

Tool is available to end users as executable versions for WinNT and Solaris. Tested platforms to date include Siemens and Agfa. The DisplayTool opening window is shown in Fig. 6.25.

Two major published standards directly relate to the topics presented in this book. One is the report of the American Association of Physicists in Medicine (AAPM) from Task Group 18. In 1999, the AAPM established a task group to recommend image quality measurement methods for gray-scale medical monitors. The task group, chaired by Dr. E. Samei, prepared a document titled, "Assessment of display performance for medical imaging systems." In it, the group presents a review of image-quality issues in gray-scale medical display devices, identifies the instrumentation needed for display performance assessment, and describes assessment methods for the different aspects of display performance in three categories: visual test methods, quantitative test methods, and advanced methods. The final document was published by AAPM in 2004.[143]

The second major standard comes out of a corresponding German effort. The German standards institution Deutsches Istitute für Normung e.V. (DIN) prepared the pre-standard DIN V 6868-57 titled, "Image quality assurance in x-ray diagnostics—Part 57: Acceptance testing for image display devices." This standard specifies requirements for acceptance testing and reference values for quality control. The test methodologies are based on SMPTE (Society of Motion Picture and TV Engineers) test patterns that define two display classes. For example, Class 1 (diagnostic) is required to have a maximum luminance of 300 cd/m^2, while the luminance with the device turned off must be less than 3.0 cd/m^2.

Another related document is the DICOM-NEMA PS 3.14, *Grayscale Display Standard Function*,[2] which aims at ensuring consistent presentation of gray-scale images across devices. Lastly, those interested in general display measurement methodologies and definitions of basic figures-of-merit in display quality should consult the Video Electronics Standards Association (VESA) *Flat-Panel Display Measurements Standard (FPDM), Version 2.0*,[58] a useful and comprehensive manual of procedures, although not specific to medical imaging applications.

Recently, the International Electrotechnical Commission (IEC) formed Working Group 62B/36 to establish a standard titled "Evaluation and routine testing in medical imaging departments – Acceptance tests – Imaging display devices." This group is tasked with preparing a document that will reflect previous work by the DIN and the AAPM report of Task Group 18.

References

[1] J. W. Allen, "Organic electroluminescence and competing technologies," *Journal of Luminescence* **60-61**, pp. 906–911 (1994).

[2] American College of Radiology/National Electrical Manufacturers Assoc. (ACR/NEMA) technical report, *Digital Imaging and Communications in Medicine (DICOM), Part 3.14, Grayscale Standard Display Function* (January 1998).

[3] V. I. Arkhipov, E. V. Emelianova, Y. H. Tak, and H. Bässler, "Charge injection into light-emitting diodes: theory and experiment," *Journal of Applied Physics* **84**, pp. 848–856 (1998).

[4] A. Badano, "Image Quality Degradation by Light Scattering Processes in High Performance Display Devices for Medical Imaging," Ph.D. thesis, University of Michigan (1999).

[5] A. Badano, "Modeling the bidirectional reflectance of emissive displays," *Applied Optics* **42(19)**, pp. 3847–3852 (2002).

[6] A. Badano, "Principles of cathode ray tube and liquid crystal display devices," *Advances in Digital Radiography: RSNA Categorical Course in Diagnostic Radiology Physics,* pp. 91–102, Radiological Society of North America, Oak Brook, IL (2003).

[7] A. Badano, S. Drilling, B. Imhoff, R. J. Jennings, R. M. Gagne, and E. Muka, "Noise in flat-panel displays with sub-pixel structure," *Medical Physics*, in press.

[8] A. Badano and M. J. Flynn, "A method for measuring veiling glare in high performance display devices," *Applied Optics* **39(13)**, pp. 2059–2066 (2000).

[9] A. Badano and M. J. Flynn, "Monte Carlo modeling of the luminance spread function in flat panel displays," *International Display Research Conference* **17**, pp. 382–385, Society for Information Display, San Jose, CA (1997).

[10] A. Badano, M. J. Flynn, and J. Kanicki, "Accurate small-spot luminance measurements," *Displays* **23**, pp. 177–182 (2002).

[11] A. Badano, M. J. Flynn, and J. Kanicki, "Small spot contrast measurements in high-performance displays," *Proc. of the 1999 SID International Symposium*, pp. 516–519 (1999).

[12] A. Badano, M. J. Flynn, S. Martin, and J. Kanicki, "Angular dependence of the luminance and contrast in medical imaging monochrome active-matrix liquid crystal displays," *Medical Physics* **30(10)**, pp. 2602–2613 (2003).

[13] A. Badano, M. J. Flynn, E. Muka, K. Compton, and T. Monsees, "Veiling glare point-spread function of medical imaging monitors," *SPIE Proc.* **3658**, pp. 458–467 (1999).

[14] A. Badano, S. J. Hipper, and R. J. Jennings, "Luminance effects on display resolution and noise," *SPIE Proc.* **4681**, pp. 305–313 (2002).

[15] A. Badano and J. Kanicki, "Characterization of crosstalk in high-resolution active-matrix liquid crystal displays for medical imaging," *SPIE Proc.* **4295**, pp. 248–253 (2001).

[16] A. Badano, S.-J. Lee, J. Kanicki, E.F. Kelley, and R.J. Jennings, "Bidirectional reflectance of organic light-emitting displays," *International Display Research Conference* **21**, pp. 21–24 (2001).

[17] M. A. Baldo, M. E. Thompson, and S. R. Forrest, "High-efficiency fluorescent organic light-emitting devices using a phosphorescent sensitizer," *Nature* **403**, pp. 750–753 (2000).

[18] P. G. J. Barten, *Contrast Sensitivity of the Human Eye and its Effect on Image Quality*, **PM 72**, SPIE Press, Bellingham, WA (1999).

[19] P. G. J. Barten, "Effects of quantization and pixel structure on the image quality of color matrix displays," *Journal of the SID* **1(2)**, pp. 147–153 (1993).

[20] P. G. J. Barten, "Physical model for the contrast sensitivity of the human eye," *SPIE Proc.* **1666**, pp. 57–72 (1992).

[21] P. G. J. Barten, "Subjective image quality of HDTV pictures," *International Display Research Conference* **19**, p. 598 (1989).

[22] B. Baxter, H. Ravindra, and R. A. Normann, "Changes in lesion detectability caused by light adaptation in retinal photoreceptors," *Investigative Radiology* **17**, pp. 394–401 (1982).

[23] D. A. Baylor and M. G. F. Fuortes, "Electrical responses of single cones in the retina of the turtle," *Journal of Physiology* **207**, pp. 77–92 (1970).

[24] M. E. Becker, "Evaluation and characterization of display reflectance," *Displays* **19**, pp. 35–54 (1998).

[25] C. Beckman, O. Nilsson, and L.-E. Paulsson, "Intraocular light scattering in vision, artistic painting, and photography," *Applied Optics* **33(21)**, pp. 4749–4753 (July 1994).

[26] M. Berggren, A. Dodabalapur, R. E. Slusher, and Z. Bao, "Light amplification in organic thin films using cascade energy transfer," *Nature* **389**, pp. 466–469 (1997).

[27] M. T. Bernius, M. Inbasekaran, J. O'Brien, and W. Wu, "Progress with light-emitting polymers," *Advanced Materials* **12(23)**, pp.1737–1750 (2000).

[28] A. Bernsten, Y. Croonen, C. Liedenbaum, H. Schoo, R. J. Visser, J. Vleggaar, et al., "Stability of polymer LEDs," *Optical Materials* **9**, pp. 125–133 (1998).

[29] A. Bernsten, P. van de Weijer, Y. Croonen, C. Liedenbaum, and J. Vleggaar, "Stability of polymer light-emitting diodes," *Philips Journal of Research* **51**, pp. 511–525 (1998).

[30] H. Blume and B. M. Hemminger, "Image presentation in digital radiology: perspectives on the emerging DICOM display function standard and its application," *Radiographics* **17**, pp. 769–777 (1997).

[31] M. Born and E. Wolf, *Principles of Optics, Third Edition*, Pergamon Press, London (1965).

[32] R. W. Boyd, *Radiometry and the Detection of Optical Radiation*, John Wiley & Sons, New York (1983).

[33] D. Braun, "Crosstalk in passive matrix polymer LED displays," *Synthetic Metals* **92**, pp. 107–113 (1998).

[34] R. Brinkley, G. Xu, A. Abileah, R. Brinkley, G. Xu, A. Abileah, et al., "Wide-viewing-angle AMLCD optimized for gray-scale operation," *Proc. of the Society for Information Display* **29**, pp. 471–474 (1998).

[35] P. L. Burn, A. B. Holmes, and A. Kraft, "Chemical tuning of electroluminescent copolymers to improve emission efficiencies and allow patterning," *Nature* **356**, pp. 47–49 (1992).

[36] J. H. Burroughes, D. D. C. Bradley, A. R. Brown, R. N. Marks, K. Mackay, R. H. Friend, et al., "Light-emitting diodes based on conjugated polymers," *Nature* **347**, pp. 539–541 (1990).

[37] P. E. Burrows, V. Bulovic, S. R. Forrest, L. S. Sapochak, D. M. McCarty, and M. E. Thompson, "Reliability and degradation of organic light emitting devices," *Applied Physics Letters* **65(23)**, pp. 2922–2924 (1994).

[38] P. E. Burrows, G. Gu, V. Bulovic, Z. Shen, S. R. Forrest, and M. E. Thompson, "Achieving full-color organic light-emitting devices for lightweight, flat-panel displays," *IEEE Transactions on Electron Devices* **44(8)**, pp. 1188–1203 (1997).

[39] P. E. Burrows, Z. Shen, and S. R. Forrest, "Saturated full color stacked organic light emitting devices," *International Display Research Conference* **17**, pp. 318–321 (1997).

[40] C. Challener, "Fast-growing polymer-OLED market is pursued by major chemical players," *Chemical Market Reporter* **258**, pp. 22–23 (2000).

[41] C.-Y. Chen and J. Kanicki, "High field-effect mobility a-Si:H TFT based on high deposition-rate PECVD materials," *IEEE Transactions on Electron Devices* **17**, pp. 437–439 (1996).

[42] J. Chen, P. J. Bos, D. R. Bryant, D. L. Johnson, S. H. Jamal, and J. R. Kelly, "Four-domain TN-LCD fabricated by reverse rubbing or double evaporation," *Proc. of the Society for Information Display* **26**, pp. 865–868 (1995).

[43] J. Chen, K.-H. Kim, J.-J. Jyu, J. H. Souk, J. R. Kelly, and P. J. Bos, "Optimum film compensation modes for TN and VA LCDs, *Proc. of the Society for Information Design 1998*, pp. 315–318 (1998).

[44] X. Cheng, Y. Hong, J. Kanicki, and L. J. Guo, "High-resolution organic polymer light-emitting pixels fabricated by imprinting technique," *J. Vac. Sci. Technol. B* **20(6)**, pp. 2877–2880 (2002).

[45] P. J. Collings, *Liquid Crystals, Nature's Delicate Phase of Matter*, A. Hilger, Bristol, England (1990).

[46] K. Compton, *Image Performance in CRT Displays,* SPIE Press, Vol. TT54, Bellingham, WA (2003).

[47] B. K. Crone, P. S. Davids, I. H. Campbell, and D. L. Smith, "Device model investigation of single layer organic light emitting diodes," *Journal of Applied Physics* **84**, pp. 833–842 (1998).

[48] S. Daly, "The visible differences predictor: an algorithm for the assessment of image fidelity," in *Digital Images and Human Vision*, Andrew B. Watson, Editor, pp. 179–206, MIT Press, Cambridge, MA (1993).

[49] R. M. A. Dawson, Z. Shen, D. A. Furst, S. Connor, J. Hsu, M. G. Kane, et al., "Design of an improved pixel for polysilicon active matrix organic LED display," *SID Tech. Dig.* **29**, pp. 11–14 (1998).

[50] R. M. A. Dawson, Z. Shen, D.A. Furst, S. Connor, J. Hsu, M.G. Kane, et al., "The impact of the transient response of organic light emitting diodes on the design of active matrix OLED displays," in *IEDM Tech. Dig.*, pp. 875–878 (1998).

[51] S. W. Depp and W. E. Howard, "Flat-panel displays," *Scientific American* **3(40)**, pp. 90–97 (March 1993).

[52] G. C. de Vries, "Contrast-enhancement under low ambient illumination," *Proc. of the Society for Information Display* **26**, pp. 32–35 (1995).

[53] P. Dyreklev, M. Berggren, O. Inganäs, M. R. Andersson, O. Wennerström, and T. Hjertberg, "Polarised electroluminescence from an oriented substituted polythiophene in a light emitting diode," *Advanced Materials* **7**, pp. 43–45 (1995).

[54] G. M. Ehemann, R. LaPeruta, and E. R. Garrity, "Method of Determining the Quality of an Aluminized, Luminescent Screen for a CRT," U.S. Patent No. 5,640,019 (1997).

[55] M. Elias, L. Simonot, and M. Menu, "Bidirectional reflectance of a diffuse background covered by a partly absorbing layer," *Optics Communications* **191**, pp. 1–7 (2001).

[56] D. Fish, N. Young, M. Childs, W. Steer, D. George, D. McCullock, et al., "A comparison of pixel circuits for active matrix polymer/organic LED displays," *SID Tech. Dig.* **33**, pp. 968–971 (2002).

[57] A. E. Flanders, R. H. Wiggins III, and M. E. Gozum, "Handheld computers in radiology," *Radiographics* **23**, pp. 1035–1047 (2003).

[58] Flat Panel Display Measurements Standard Working Group, Video Electronics Standards Association (VESA), *Flat Panel Display Measurements Standard, Version 2.0* (May 2003).

[59] M. J. Flynn, DisplayTool software, available upon request to mikef@rad.hfh.edu.

[60] M. J. Flynn and A. Badano, "Image quality degradation by light scattering in display devices," *Journal of Digital Imaging* **12(2)**, pp. 50–59 (May 1999).

[61] M. J. Flynn, Jerzy Kanicki, Aldo Badano, and William R. Eyler, "High-fidelity electronic display of digital radiographs," *Radiographics* **19(6)**, pp. 1653–1669 (1999).

[62] M. J. Flynn, T. McDonald, E. G. DiBello, J. L. Jorgensen, and W. Worobey, "Flat panel display technology for high performance radiographic imaging," *SPIE Proc.* **2431**, pp. 360–371 (1995).

[63] S. R. Forrest, P. E. Burrows, Z. Shen, G. Gu, V. Bulovic, and M. E. Thompson, "The stacked OLED (SOLED): a new type of organic device for achieving high-resolution full-color displays," *Synthetic Metals* **91**, pp. 9–13 (1997).

[64] S. R. Forrest, P. E. Burrows, and M. E. Thompson, "The dawn of organic electronics," *IEEE Spectrum* **37(8)**, pp. 29–34 (2000).

[65] R. H. Fowler and L. Nordheim, "Electron emission in intense electric fields," *Proc. Roy. Soc. London* **119A**, pp. 173–181 (1928).

[66] M. Fujihira, L. M. Do, A. Koike, and E. M. Han, "Growth of dark spots by interdiffusion across organic layers in organic electroluminescent devices," *Applied Physics Letters* **68(13)**, pp. 1787–1789 (1996).

[67] Y. Fukuda, T. Watanabe, T. Wakimoto, S. Miyaguchi, and M. Tsuchida, "An organic LED display exhibiting pure RGB colors," *Synthetic Metals* **111-112**, pp. 1–6 (2000).

[68] R. E. Gill, P. van de Weijer, C. T. H. Liedenbaum, H. F. M. Schoo, A. Berntsen, J. J. M. Vleggaar, et al., "Stability and characterization of large area polymer light-emitting diodes over extended periods," *Optical Materials* **12(2-3)**, pp. 183–187 (1999).

[69] N. C. Greenham, S. C. Moratti, D. D. C. Bradley, R. H. Friend, and A. B. Holmes, "Efficient light-emitting diodes based on polymers with high electron affinities," *Nature* **365**, pp. 628–630 (1993).

[70] G. Gu and S. R. Forrest, "Design of flat-panel displays based on organic light-emitting devices," *IEEE Journal on Selected Topics in Quantum Electronics* **4(1)**, pp. 83–99 (1998).

[71] R. W. Gymer, "Organic electroluminescent displays," *Endeavour* **20**, pp. 115–120 (1996).

[72] M. Hack, R. Kwong, M. S. Weaver, M. Lu, and J. J. Brown, "Active-matrix technology for high efficiency OLED displays," in *Proc. of IDMC '02*, pp. 57–60 (2002).

[73] T. B. Harvey III, Q. Shi, and F. So, "Passivated Organic Device having Alternating Layers of Polymer and Dielectric," U.S. Patent No. 5,757,126 (May 1998).

[74] F. Hasselbach and H.-R. Krauss, "Backscattered electrons and their influence on contrast in the scanning electron microscope," *Scanning Microscopy* **2(2)**, pp. 1947–1956 (1988).

[75] Y. He, "Polyfluorene Light-Emitting Devices and a-Si:H TFT Pixel Circuits for Active-Matrix Organic Light Emitting Displays," Ph.D. thesis, University of Michigan (2000).

[76] Y. He, S. Gong, R. Hattori, and J. Kanicki, "High performance organic polymer light-emitting heterostructure devices," *Applied Physics Letters* **74**, pp. 2265–2267 (1999).

[77] Y. He, R. Hattori, and J. Kanicki, "Current-source a-Si:H thin-film transistor circuit for active-matrix organic light-emitting displays," *IEEE Electron Device Letters* **21(12)**, pp. 590–592 (2000).

[78] Y. He, R. Hattori, and J. Kanicki, "Improved a-Si:H TFT pixel electrode circuits for active-matrix organic light emitting displays," *IEEE Transactions on Electron Devices* **48(7)**, pp. 1322–1325 (2001).

[79] S. Hecht and Y. Hsia, "Dark adaptation following light adaptation to red and white lights," *Journal of the Optical Society of America* **35(4)**, pp. 261–267 (April 1945).

[80] S. Hecht and Y. Hsia, "Relation between visual acuity and illumination," *Journal of General Physiology* **11**, pp. 255–281 (1928).

[81] P. K. H. Ho, J.-S. Kim, J. H. Burroughes, H. Becker, S. F. Y. Li, T. M. Brown, et al., "Molecular-scale interface engineering for polymer light-emitting diodes," *Nature* **404**, pp. 481–484 (2000).

[82] C. D. Hoke, H. Mori, and P. J. Bos, "An ultra-wide-viewing angle STNLCD with a negative-birefringence compensation film," *International Display Research Conference* **17**, pp. 21–24 (1997).

[83] Y. Hong, J. Kanicki, and R. Hattori, "Novel poly-Si TFT pixel electrode circuits and current programmed active-matrix driving methods for AM-OLED," *SID Tech. Dig.* **33**, pp. 618–621 (2002).

[84] Y. Hong, J.-Y. Nahm, and J. Kanicki, "100 dpi 4-a-Si:H TFTs active-matrix organic polymer light-emitting display," *IEEE Journal of Selected Topics in Quantum Electronics* **10**, pp. 16–25 (2004).

[85] Y. Hong, J.-Y. Nahm, and J. Kanicki, "Optoelectrical properties of four amorphous silicon thin-film transistors 200 dpi active-matrix organic polymer light-emitting display," *Applied Physics Letters* **83(16)**, pp. 3233–3235 (2003).

[86] Y. Hong, J.-Y. Nahm, and J. Kanicki, "200 dpi 4-a-Si:H TFTs current-driven AM-PLEDs," *SID '03 Digest,* pp. 22–25 (2003).

[87] ISO Technical Report 9241-7, *Ergonomic Requirements for Office Work with Visual Display Terminals* (1997).

[88] G. E. Jabbour, S. E. Shaheen, M. M. Morrell, B. Kippelen, N. R. Armstrong, and N. Peyghambarian, "Aluminum composite cathodes: a new method for the fabrication of efficient and bright organic light-emitting devices," *Optics and Photonics News* **10(4)**, p. 24 (1999).

[89] Y.-C. Jeong, C.-C. Park, and L.-S. Kim, "A new crosstalk compensation method in line inversion TFT-LCDs," *IEEE Transactions on Systems and Circuits,* **44(6)**, pp. 552–555 (1997).

[90] G. R. Jones, E. F. Kelley, and T. A. Germer, "Specular and diffuse reflection measurements of electronic displays," *Proc. of the Society for Information Display* **27**, pp. 203–206 (1996).

[91] G. W. Jones, W. E. Howard, and S. M. Zimmerman, "Sealing structure for organic light emitting devices," U.S. Patent No. 6,198,220 B1 (2001).

[92] E. Kaneko, *Liquid Crystal TV Display: Principles and Applications of Liquid Crystal Displays*, KTK Scientific Publishers, Tokyo (1987).

[93] J. Kanicki, Y. He, and R. Hattori, "a-Si:H pixel electrode circuits for AM-OLEDs," *SPIE Proc.* 4295, pp. 147–158 (2001).

[94] J. Kanicki, J. Lan, A. Catalano, J. Keane, W. Den Boer, and T. Gu, "Patterning of transparent conductive oxide thin films by wet etching for a-Si:H TFT-LCDs," *Journal of Electronic Materials* 25, pp. 1806–1817 (1996).

[95] M. Kawasaki, N. Tani, and R. Onishi, "Improvement of contrast and brightness by using crystal pigment phosphor screens," *Proc. of the Society for Information Display* 29, pp. 266–269 (1998).

[96] P. A. Keller, *The Cathode-Ray Tube: Technology, History and Applications*, Palisades Press, New York (1992).

[97] E. F. Kelley, "Display reflectance model based on BRDF," *Displays* 19, pp. 27–34 (1998).

[98] J. Kido, K. Masato, and N. Katsutoshi, "Multilayer white light-emitting organic electroluminescent device," *Science* 267, pp. 1132–1334 (March 1995).

[99] J. H. Kim, Y. Hong, and J. Kanicki, "Amorphous silicon thin-film transistors-based organic polymer light-emitting displays," *IEEE Electron Device Letters* 24(7), pp. 451–453 (2003).

[100] M. Kimura, I. Yudasaka, S. Kanbe, H. Kobayashi, H. Kiguchi, S. Seki, et al., "Low-temperature polysilicon thin-film transistor driving with integrated driver for high-resoluition light emitting polymer display," *IEEE Trans. Electron Devices* 46(12), pp. 2282–2288 (1999).

[101] Kodak, "Kodak, Sanyo unveil 15-inch flat-panel display," http://wwwnl.kodak.com/US/en/corp/display/sanyoFlat.jhtml, Chiba, Japan, posted October 2, 2002.

[102] K. Kohm, "Visual CRT sharpness estimation using a fiducial marker set," *SPIE Proc.* 4319, pp. 286–297 (2001).

[103] H. Kubota, S. Miyaguchi, S. Ishizuka, T. Wakimoto, J. Funaki, Y. Fukuda, et al., "Organic LED full color passive-matrix display," *Journal of Luminescence* 87-89, pp. 56–60 (2000).

[104] J.-H. Lan and J. Kanicki, "Planarized copper-gate hydrogenated amorphous silicon thin-film transistors for active-matrix liquid crystal displays," *IEEE Transactions on Electron Devices* 20(3), p. 129 (1999).

[105] S. Lee, A. Badano, and J. Kanicki, "Monte Carlo modeling of organic polymer light-emitting devices on flexible plastic substrates," *SPIE Proc.* 4800, pp. 156–163 (2002).

[106] G. Leising, S. Tasch, F. Meghdadi, L. Athouel, G. Froyer, and U. Scherf, "Blue electroluminescence with ladder-type poly(para-phenylene) and parahexaphenyl," *Synthetic Metals* 81, pp. 185–189 (1996).

[107] X. C. Li, F. Cacialli, M. Giles, J. Gruner, R. H. Friend, A. B. Holmes, et al., "Light-emitting-diodes based on Poly(Methacrylate)s with distyrylbenzene and oxadiazole side-chains," *Advanced Materials* 7, pp. 898–900 (1995).

[108] F. R. Libsch and A. Lien, "A compensation driving method for reducing crosstalk in XGA and higher-resolution TFT-LCDs," *Proc. of the Society for Information Display* **26**, pp. 253–256 (1995).

[109] F. R. Libsch and A. Lien, "Understanding crosstalk in high-resolution color thin-film-transistor liquid crystal displays," *IBM Journal of Research and Development* **42(3/4)**, pp. 467–479 (May 1998).

[110] J.-J. Lih, C-F Sung, M. S. Weaver, M. Hack, and J. J. Brown, "A phosphorescent active-matrix OLED display driven by amorphous silicon backplane," *SID Tech. Dig.* **34**, pp. 14–17 (2003).

[111] S. F. Lim, K. Ke, W. Wang, and S. J. Chua, "Correlation between dark spot growth and pinhole size in organic light-emitting diodes," *Applied Physics Letters* **78**, pp. 2116–2118 (2001).

[112] M. Lindfors, "Accuracy and repeatability of the ISO 9241-7 test method," *Displays* **19**, pp. 3–16 (1998).

[113] C. J. Lloyd, M. Mizukami, and P. R. Boyce, "A preliminary model of lightning display interaction," *Journal of the Illuminating Engineering Society* **25(2)**, pp. 59–69 (1996).

[114] J. R. Mansell and A. W. Woodhead, "Contrast loss in image devices due to electrons back-scattered from the fluorescent screen," *Journal of Physics D: Applied Physics* **16**, pp. 2269–2278 (1983).

[115] S. Martin, A. Badano, and J. Kanicki, "Characterization of a high quality monochrome AM-LCD monitor for digital radiology," *SPIE Proc.* **4681**, pp. 293–304 (2002).

[116] Y. Masutani, S. Tahata, M. Hayashi, T. Onawa, K. Kobayashi, K. Nagata, et al., "Novel TFT-array structure for LCD monitors with in-plane switching mode," *Proc. of the Society for Information Display* **28**, pp. 15–18 (1997).

[117] J. McElvain, H. Antoniadis, M. R. Hueschen, J. N. Miller, D. M. Roitman, J. R. Sheats, et al., "Formation and growth of black spots in organic light-emitting diodes," *Journal of Applied Physics* **80**, pp. 6002–6007 (1996).

[118] Z. Meng and M. Wong, "Active-matrix organic light-emitting diode displays realized using metal-induced unilaterally crystallized polycrystalline silicon thin-film transistors," *IEEE Trans. Electron Devices* **49(6)**, pp. 991–996 (2002).

[119] D. Mentley, *Flat Panel Display Market Overview*, iSuppli/Stanford Resources (2002).

[120] D. E. Mentley, "State of flat-panel display technology and future trends," *Proc. of the IEEE* **90(4)**, pp. 453–459 (2002).

[121] A. A. Michelson, *Studies in Optics*, The University of Chicago Press, Chicago (1962).

[122] I. S. Millard, "High-efficiency polyfluorene polymers suitable for RGB applications," *Synthetic Metals* **111-112**, pp. 119–123 (2000).

[123] H. Mori and P. J. Bos, "Application of a negative birefringence film to various LCD modes," *International Display Research Conference* **17**, pp. M88–M97 (1997).

[124] E. Muka, T. Mertelmeier, and R. M. Slone, "Impact of phosphor luminance noise on the specification of high-resolution CRT displays for medical imaging," *SPIE Proc.* **3031**, pp. 210–221 (1997).

[125] S. Musa, "Active-matrix liquid-crystal displays," *Scientific American* **277**, pp. 87–92 (1997).

[126] M. S. Nam, J. W. Wu, Y. J. Choi, K. H. Yoon, J. H. Jung, J. Y. Kim, et al., "Wide-viewing-angle TFT-LCD with photoaligned four-domain TN mode," *Proc. of the Society for Information Display* **28**, pp. 933–936 (1997).

[127] J. A. Nichols, T. N. Jackson, M. H. Lu, and M. Hack, "a-Si:H TFT active-matrix phosphorescent OLED pixel," *SID Tech. Dig.* **33**, pp. 1368–1371 (2002).

[128] R. A. Norman, B. S. Baxter, and H. Ravindra, "Photoreceptor contributions to contrast sensitivity: Applications in radiological diagnosis," *IEEE Transactions on Systems, Man, and Cybernetics* **SMC-13(5)**, pp. 944–953 (1983).

[129] R. A. Norman and I. Perlman, "The effects of background illumination on the photoresponses of red and green cones," *Journal of General Physiology* **286**, pp. 491–507 (1979).

[130] R. A. Norman and F. S. Werblin, "Control of retinal sensitivity: light and dark adaptation of vertebrate rods and cones," *Journal of General Physiology* **63**, pp. 37–61 (1974).

[131] K. Ohmuro, S. Kataoka, T. Sasaki, and Y. Koike, "Development of super-high-image-quality vertical-alignment-mode LCD," *Proc. of the Society for Information Display* **28**, pp. 845–848 (1997).

[132] M. Ohta, H. Tsutsu, H. Takahara, I. Kobayashi, T. Uemura, and Y. Takubo, "A novel current programmed pixel for active matrix OLED displays," *SID Tech. Dig.* **34**, pp. 108–111 (2003).

[133] Y. Ono, Y. Ohtani, K. Hiratsuka, and T. Morimoto, "A new antireflective and antistatic double-layered coating for CRTs," *Proc. of the Society for Information Display* **23**, pp. 511–514 (1992).

[134] L. Ozawa, *Cathodoluminescence: Theory and Applications*, Kodansha, Tokyo (1990).

[135] E. Peli, J. Yang, R. Goldstein, and A. Reeves, "Effect of luminance on suprathreshold contrast perception," *Journal of the Optical Society of America A* **8**, pp. 1352–1359 (August 1991).

[136] M. Pope, H. Kallmann, and P. Magnante, "Electroluminescence in organic crystals," *Journal of Chem. Phys.* **38**, pp. 2042–2048 (1963).

[137] D. A. Reimann, M. J. Flynn, and J. J. Ciarelli, "System to maintain perceptually linear networked display devices," *SPIE Proc.* **2431**, pp. 316–326 (1995).

[138] O. W. Richardson, "On the negative radiation from hot platinum," *Proc. Camb. Phil. Soc.* **11**, p. 286 (1902).

[139] G. G. Roberts, M. McGinnity, W. A. Barlow, and P. S. Vincett, "Electroluminescence, photoluminescence and electroabsorption of a lightly substituted anthracene langmuir film," *Solid State Communications* **32**, pp. 683–686 (1979).

[140] J. W. Roberts and E. F. Kelley, "Measurements of static noise in display images," *SPIE Proc.* **4295**, pp. 211–218 (2001).

[141] S. P. Rogers, "Organic Electroluminescent Device Hermetic Encapsulation Package and Method of Fabrication," U.S. Patent No. 5,874,804 (1999).

[142] B. E. A. Saleh and K. Lu, "The Fourier scope: An optical instrument for measuring LCD viewing-angle characteristics," *Journal of the SID* **4(1)**, pp. 33–40 (1996).

[143] E. Samei, A. Badano, D. Chakraborty, K. Compton, C. Cornelius, K. Corrigan, et al., *Assessment of Display Performance for Medical Imaging Systems*, draft report of the American Association of Physicists in Medicine Task Group 18, Version 9.1 (2003).

[144] E. Samei and M. J. Flynn, "A method for in-field evaluation of the modulation transfer function of electronic display devices," *SPIE Proc.* **4319**, pp. 599–607 (2001).

[145] Samsung SDI Co., "SDI develops ultra fine high-speed LCD for handset," http://www.samsungsdi.co.kr (in Japanese and English), posted July 30, 2003.

[146] J. L. Sanford and F. R. Libsch, "TFT AMOLED pixel circuits and driving methods," *SID Tech. Dig.* **34**, pp. 10–13 (2003).

[147] T. Sasaoka, M. Sekiya, A. Yumoto, J. Yamada, T. Hirano, Y. Iwase, et al., "A 13.0-inch AM-OLED display with top emitting structure and adaptive current mode programmed pixel circuit (TAC)," *SID Tech. Dig.* **32**, pp.384–387 (2001).

[148] W. Schottky and J. Issendorff, "Quasineutrale elektrische diffusion im ruhenden und strömenden gas," *Zeitshrift für Physik* **31**, pp. 163–201 (1925).

[149] M. I. Sezan, K. L. Yip, and S. J. Daly, "Uniform perceptual quantization: applications to digital radiology," *IEEE Transactions on Systems, Man, and Cybernetics* **SMC-17(4)**, pp. 622–634 (1987).

[150] T. Shimoda, M. Kimura, S. Seki, H. Kobayashi, S. Kanbe, S. Miyashita, et al., "Technology for active matrix light emitting polymer displays," in *Proc. IEDM '99*, pp. 107–110 (1999).

[151] T. Shimoda, H. Ohshima, S. Miyashita, M. Kimura, T. Ozawa, I. Yudasaka, et al., "High resolution light emitting polymer display driven by low temperature polysilicon thin film transistor with integrated driver," *Proc. Asia Display '98*, pp. 217–220 (1998).

[152] G. Spencer, P. Shirley, K. Zimmerman, and D. P. Greenberg, "Physically based glare effects for digital images," in *Computer Graphics Proceedings, Annual Conference Series SIGGRAPH 95*, pp. 325–334 (1995).

[153] W. S. Stiles, "The effect of glare on the brightness difference threshold," *Proc. Royal Soc. London* **B104**, pp. 322–351 (1929).

[154] W. S. Stiles and B. H. Crawford, "The luminous efficiency of rays entering the eye pupil at different points," *Proc. Royal Soc. London* **122**, pp. 428–450 (1937).

[155] C. W. Tang and S. A. Van Slyke, "Organic electroluminescent diodes," *Applied Physics Letters* **51(12)**, pp. 913–915 (September 1987).

[156] S. Terada, G. Izumi, Y. Sato, M. Takahashi, M. Tada, K. Kawase, et al., "A 24-inch AM-OLED display with XGA resolution by novel seamless tiling technology," *SID Tech. Dig.* **34**, pp. 1463–1465 (2003).

[157] H. S. Tong and G. Prando, "Hygroscopic ion-induced antiglare/antistatic coating for CRT applications," *Proc. of the Society for Information Display* **23**, pp. 514–517 (1992).

[158] Toshiba Matsushita Display Technology Co., Ltd., "Toshiba Matsushita Display Technology introduces world's largest polymer organic light-emitting diode display," http://www.tmdisplay.com/tm_dsp/press/2002/04-16a.htm, posted April 16, 2002.

[159] T. Tsujimura, Y. Kobayashi, K. Murayama, A. Tanaka, M. Morooka, E. Fukumoto, et al., "A 20-inch OLED display driven by super-amorphous-silicon technology," *SID Tech. Dig.* **34**, pp. 6–9 (2003).

[160] N. Umezu, Y. Nakano, T. Sakai, R. Yoshitake, W. Herlitschke, and S. Kubota, "Specular and diffuse reflection measurement feasibility study of ISO 9241, part 7: method," *Displays* **19**, pp. 17–25 (1998).

[161] J. J. van Oekel, "Improving the contrast of CRTs under low ambient illumination with a graphite coating," *Proc. of the Society for Information Display* **26**, pp. 427–430 (1995).

[162] J. J. van Oekel, M. J. Severens, G. M. H. Timmermans, and A. A. M. Mouws, "Improving contrast and color saturation of CRTs by Al_2O_3 shadow mask coating, *Proc. of the Society for Information Display* **28**, pp. 436–439 (1997).

[163] P. S. Vincett, W. A. Barlow, R. A. Hann, and G. G. Roberts, "Electrical conduction and low voltage blue electroluminescence in vacuum-deposited organic films," *Thin Solid Films* **94**, pp. 171–183 (1982).

[164] H. Wakemoto, S. Asada, N. Kato, Y. Yamamoto, M. Tsukane, T. Tsurugi, et al., "An advanced in-plane switching mode TFT-LCD," *Proc. of the Society for Information Display* **26**, pp. 929–932 (1997).

[165] M. Weibrecht, G. Spekowius, P. Quadflieg, et al., "Image quality assessment of monochrome monitors for medical soft copy displays," *SPIE Proc.* **3031**, pp. 232–244 (1997).

[166] S. L. Wright, S. Millman, and M. Kodate, "Measurement and digital compensation of crosstalk and photoleakage in high-resolution TFTLCDs," *SPIE Proc.* **3636**, pp. 200–211 (1999).

[167] N. Yamada, S. Kohzaki, F. Funada, and K. Awane, "A full-color video-rate anti-ferroelectric LCD with wide viewing angle," *Proc. of the Society for Information Display* **17**, pp. 789–792 (1995).

[168] Y. Yang and S. C. Chang, "Pyramid-shaped pixels for full-color organic emissive displays," *Applied Physics Letters* **77(7)**, pp. 936–938 (2000).

[169] G. Yu, H. Nishino, A. J. Heeger, T. A. Chen, and R. D. Rieke, "Enhanced electroluminescence from semiconducting polymer blends," *Synthetic Metals* **72**, pp. 249–252 (1995).

[170] C. Zhang, H. Von Seggern, B. Kraabel, H. W. Schmidt, and A. J. Heeger, "Blue emission from polymer light-emitting diodes using non-conjugated polymer blends with air-stable electrodes," *Synthetic Metals* **72**, pp. 185–188 (1995).

[171] K. Ziemelis, "Display technology: glowing developments," *Nature* **399**, pp. 408–411 (2000).

[172] S. M. Zimmerman, G. W. Jones, and H. E. Webster, "Sealing Structure for Organic Light Emitting Devices," U.S. Patent No. 6,198,220 (May 2001).

Index

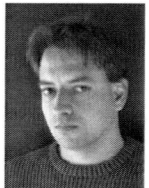

Aldo Badano received his Ph.D. degree in Nuclear Engineering from the University of Michigan in 1999. He is currently a research scientist with the Division of Imaging and Applied Mathematics, Office of Science and Engineering Laboratories, Center for Devices and Radiological Health, at the U.S. Food and Drug Administration, where he leads a research program on the evaluation of medical displays. Dr. Badano's research focuses on the objective assessment of image quality in medical imaging sensors and image display devices using advanced experimental and computational methods. He is a referee for several scientific journals and a reviewer of technical grants for the U.S. Department of Defense and the National Institutes of Health. He has authored or coauthored more than 60 publications. He is a member of SID, AAPM, and SPIE.

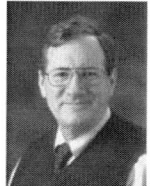

Michael Flynn obtained his Ph.D. in Nuclear Science from the University of Michigan in 1975. He is presently a Senior Scientist at Henry Ford Health System in Detroit, Michigan, where he conducts sponsored research on medical display, digital radiography, and computed tomography. Currently an Adjunct Professor of Nuclear Engineering and Radiological Science at the University of Michigan, Dr. Flynn has taught a graduate course on radiation imaging for over 20 years. His scientific work emphasizes the importance of high-fidelity display to complete the medical imaging process.

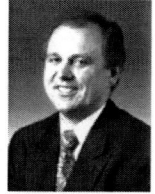

Jerzy Kanicki received his Ph.D. degree in Sciences (D.Sc.) from the Universite Libre de Bruxeles (Belgium) in 1982. He subsequently became a Research Staff Member at the IBM Thomas J. Watson Research Center in Yorktown Heights, New York, working on hydrogenated amorphous silicon devices for photo-voltaic and flat-panel display applications. In 1994 he moved to the University of Michigan as a Professor in the Department of Electrical Engineering and Computer Science, where he did leading work on various flat-panel display technologies until 2000. Since 2000 he has worked on a variety of fundamental problems related to organic and molecular electronics. In 2002–2003 he spent a sabbatical year at the Center for Polymers and Organic Solids, University of California-Santa Barbara, conducting research in the area of conducting polymer devices. Dr. Kanicki is the author or coauthor of over 250 publications in journals and conference proceedings, and he has edited two books and three conference proceedings. He has presented numerous invited talks at national and international meetings in the area of organic and inorganic semiconductor devices. More information about his research group activities can be found at www.eecs.umich.edu/omelab/.